WOW!

YOU LOOK

FANTASTIC

Your Journey to a Happier, Healthier Life

Nancy N. Wilson

Publisher's Notes

WOW! You Look Fantastic!

Your Journey to a Happier, Healthier Life
By Nancy N. Wilson

© Blurtigo Holdings, LLC
1st Edition – February 2019
Published in the United States of America
ISBN: 9781797425313

Cover Image 485630253@iStock.com

Disclaimer and Terms of Use:

The Author and Publisher have strived to be as accurate and complete as possible in the creation of this book. While all attempts have been made to verify information provided in this publication, the Author and Publisher assume no responsibility for errors, omissions, or contrary interpretation of the subject matter herein. Perceived slights of specific persons, peoples, or organizations are unintentional.

The information in this book is not a substitute for licensed professionals who can diagnose, treat, and give medical advice. If you do anything I recommend without the supervision of a licensed medical doctor, you do so at your own risk.

This information is for educational purposes only. It is not intended to be a substitute for professional medical advice and should not be relied on as health or personal advice. The author is not trying to prescribe any medical treatment since under the laws of the United States only a licensed medical doctor (an MD) can do so.

Never disregard the advice of a medical professional or delay in seeking it because of something you have read in this book. You and only you are responsible if you choose to do anything based on the information in this book. Do not embark on any new diet or exercise program without first consulting with your physician.

Dedication

To everyone who wants to live a happier, healthier life. I hope that you will choose to take this journey with me!

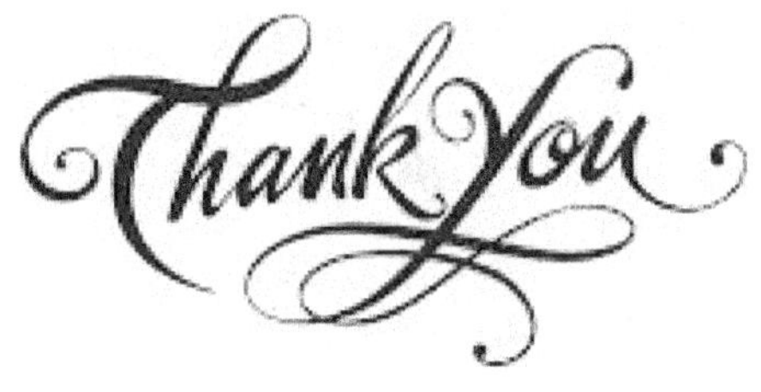

... for buying my book.
If you enjoy it, please take a minute
and post a review on the platform where
you made your purchase

WOW! You Look Fantastic!

Your Journey to a Happier, Healthier Life

For a complete list of my published books,
please, visit my websites
https://www.nancynwilson.com
https://www.mamaslegacycookbooks.com

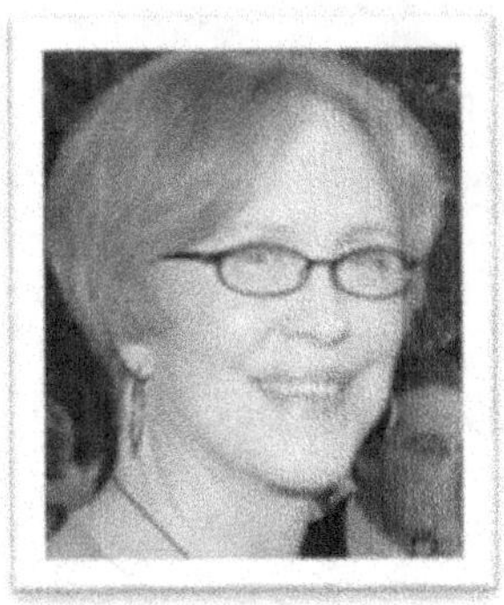

Nancy N. Wilson

Table of Contents

Introduction

Welcome to ***WOW! You Look Fantastic!*** This subject is my passion, one that has developed over a very long lifetime. I was fortunate to have inherited a wonderful gene pool that included height, a slender frame, high energy, and extremely good health.

For most of my life , I was diligent in the care of my body. I hate to admit that after my divorce at age 42, my good health practices became erratic. Until then, I had planned, prepared, and eaten well-balanced meals, exercised regularly, never consumed caffeine or alcohol and did not smoke.

As a healthy way of life – that is a good plan, which served me well over the years, but little by little, things began to change.

I started drinking multiple cans of coke daily – or more explicitly – TAB (so a double hit on my body, caffeine *and* artificial sweetener). Fast food became a regular part of my diet, and eventually, I began smoking and started drinking wine. I thought I had entered the world of sophisticated people.

I'm happy to say that my exercise regimen remained constant – aerobics, Jazzercize, and social swing dancing were important activities for me over the years. Plus, when I moved to Manhattan, walking was also part of my daily routine.

So, where was the problem? Simple – my other healthy practices were inconsistent. My focus was on taking care of four children as a single mom, running my interior design business, and socializing.

I was a young, reasonably good-looking single woman who didn't want to be alone the rest of my life. Finding someone to love was a major goal –

and I thought it was important to put myself "out there" and look good in the process (which was the driver for the exercise).

When you throw into the mix the problem that I am a stress eater – and what I eat under stress is not healthy (favorites are ice cream, pastries, chocolate, diet coke, and Frappuccinos), my overall lifestyle was rapidly deteriorating to extremely unhealthy.

For the first time in my life, I gained a little weight and began yo-yo dieting. My weight which had been between 130 - 140 pounds on my 5'9" frame for most of my life began to increase. I would realize the gain and lose the weight for a while – then, I would gain it back, plus more.

I tried Atkins, which my body doesn't tolerate well. I tried all the fad diets of the time: Grapefruit Diet, Cabbage Soup Diet, appetite suppressants (Ayds, Dexetrim, and Ephedra – all three were eventually taken off the market), SlimFast, Scarsdale Diet, and, of course, Weight Watchers.

They all worked when I worked them, but none gave me the lifelong change I was looking for – and needed. The weight continued to yo-yo.

In 2010 some personal challenges took all my focus and energy with nothing left for self-care and healthy eating. In 2012, when my son died, the stress eating flew out of control. I stopped exercising and started to gain weight – pound after pound.

The unhealthy eating and weight gain continued for the next five years because I was in too much mental and emotional pain to pay attention.

Then, one morning in early January 2018, I stepped on the scales and saw ***203.8 pounds – almost 64 lbs. over my lifetime standard of 140 lbs.*** That was it! It had to stop!

I did not want to live my life overweight and at risk for serious health problems. Not only was I extremely overweight (borderline obese), my mother had developed Type 2 diabetes in her 70s and I could see myself following in her footsteps. In my mind, there was no choice but to change the way I had been living for the past eight years.

The irony in this story is that I had been writing a blog for over two years that was focused on clean eating and good health. I believed everything I had written; but, I had not been following my own advice.

I had done a lot of research for my blog and was very clear about all the things I was doing that were harmful to my well-being. I knew exactly what I needed to change in order to create the lifestyle I wanted for the rest of my life. BUT . . . I wasn't doing any of it. Anger, overwhelming grief, sadness, frustration, and more were ruling my life, and I was accepting it.

I admit I was so desperate when I saw "203.8 lbs." on the scale that I opted for **Nutrisystem** as a starting point. I needed something to happen fast – and I needed it RIGHT NOW.

It worked. In the first month, I lost 10 lbs. but, one month was all I could tolerate. I got sick of the food very quickly; and, much to my surprise there were a lot of additives in the food that I did not like putting into my body. Plus, it was expensive. So, I did not continue down that path.

I am not sorry that I started with Nutrisystem. It was a desperately needed kickstart to losing weight. It also taught me a valuable lesson – **portion control**.

When I received my first shipment and started eating the meals, I was surprised at how small the portions were – and yet, it was enough. I was never hungry and I started losing weight. I was careful and followed the instructions exactly. In other words, I worked the program – and it worked for me.

When I decided not to continue with the system, I knew I had to find another way to lose weight. Giving up was not an option. I was determined to stay on track and get back to a healthy weight. It was clear that another change was necessary.

I finally accepted that reaching my goal wasn't going to be easy. I realized that ***it would take as long as it would take***. Even though I was not thrilled with that realization, I made my peace with it and continued to move forward.

There is another twist to this story that you should know.

I started Nutrisystem on January 29. Four weeks later as I was finishing up the first month of "dieting," I began suffering from agonizing back pain. After two weeks of misdiagnoses, I ended up in the E.R. with the diagnosis of a cracked vertebrae.

I was immediately hospitalized. The first thing they did (after administering morphine for the pain) was to put me in a body brace. Four days later they transferred me to a skilled nursing facility for 3½ weeks where I was given more pain pills than I care to think about and struggled through daily rehab to get back on my feet and walking again.

This was the perfect excuse to forget about losing weight and eat whatever I wanted. But, to my own amazement, I chose not to do that. I was determined to stay on my journey back to eating well and living well.

Fortunately, the facility had an excellent meal service (with good food). I watched my portions carefully and continued to count calories – and it worked.

It not only worked, it also set the path that I would follow from that point on.

Which brings us to the present – ***one year later.***

I have recovered completely from my injury and I have returned to work. I have gradually rebuilt my stamina through walking – starting out with a few steps a day and building up to 4000+ steps a day. I have lost 40 pounds and still losing – moving slowly toward my target weight of 150 pounds.

It has been a long, slow process, but I'm OK with that for several reasons:
1. It has allowed my body to adjust to the change and I feel great.
2. I will be able to keep the weight off because I have a completely new way of eating.
3. I do not have huge flabs of skin that often result from extreme, fast weight loss.
4. I started the journey knowing it would take time – my expectations were set appropriately from the beginning.

This book summarizes the information I gathered and applied during my journey. I can promise you, from personal experience, that this is the way to a healthy weight and a healthy life for the rest of your life.

Chapter One
Faulty Strategies

Yo-Yo Dieting

This is an appropriate name for a phenomenon that many of us know far too well!

When your focus is continuously on losing weight, you start every new fad diet with great enthusiasm and do well for a while. You lose a few pounds – often quicker than you expected. But . . . at some point, your determination begins to falter and the weight begins to reappear – sometimes slowly and sometimes quickly.

The most frustrating part is that you often end up weighing more than you did when you started the diet. OUCH!

Finally, you are forced to acknowledge defeat and quickly slip back into your old eating habits. You continue to struggle with the desire to lose weight and eventually you look for another diet to help you – and, so, the yo-yo begins, again.

Extreme Eating

If you look at all the diets you have tried in the past, my guess is that they cover the full spectrum of diet possibilities – from eating only a select number of foods for a certain period-of-time to the elimination of whole food groups (even healthy foods like fruits and vegetables).

Extreme eating patterns and severely restrictive diets of any kind are not good for your body or your general health. They make great promises; but, set you up for failure because they are always short-term fixes. They cannot be sustained over an extended period of time.

When you start tallying up how many days you "have to be on a new diet to lose X-number of pounds," it is a sure indication to steer clear immediately! If you continue, you can be certain that any pounds you lose will be regained once you go off the diet.

Most fad diets are not enjoyable, not good for your health, and certainly not sustainable for long. Eventually, you will return to "real life" and most people immediately fall back into old eating habits and the weight returns.

For a diet to be successful in terms of weight loss and a healthier body, you need to learn how to **_eat for life_**, not for 30 days or eight weeks.

A Dieting Mindset

Living your life thinking about dieting, talking about dieting, and planning your life around dieting is not a pleasant way to live. In fact, it makes you miserable.

Life should be about enjoying time with friends and family; preparing and consuming delicious, healthy meals; refreshing yourself through your favorite activities; and experiencing success in your professional life.

It should not be spent obsessing about the way you look, the food you are eating (or not eating), the extra pounds you are carrying, and constantly on the lookout for a new and better way to change your body.

Life should be enjoyed pursuing things that make you feel good – living a healthy lifestyle that delivers total wellness, including mental happiness. A dieting mindset does not fit into that picture.

People with a dieting mindset tend to do the following things:

1. **They talk about dieting all the time** – what they are planning to do, what they are doing, what they did, and where they failed.

2. **They become critical of friends and family who are not following the same regimen** – misery loves company.

3. **They focus on what they are doing wrong** – continually beating themselves up for every slip (major or minor), or when another diet fails.

Living with that mindset is stressful and exhausting – mentally and physically. Your body is forced to continually adjust to a new eating and/or starving mode, which forces you to mentally jump back and forth from happy anticipation of the "new you" when you are losing weight – to feeling like a failure and losing confidence when the diet fails, once again. It is all too much!

Set Yourself Free

If any of the above strategies sound familiar, you may be one of the many who joins Sisyphus in his sorrow. He was forced to deal with the unspeakable penalty of pushing the rock to the top of the hill – exerting his whole being in the process, only for it to roll down the hill again.

Unlike Sisyphus, you do not have to repeat the same discouraging uphill battle you have been fighting for years.

In her book, *Why Diets Make Us Fat*, neuroscientist **_Sandra Aamodt_** tackles why traditional diets don't work for many people, and often leave the dieter worse off than before.

She explains her philosophy of ***mindful eating,*** which is, "...eating with attention and joy, without judgment. That ***includes attention to hunger*** *and fullness, to the experience of eating and to its effects on our bodies."*

Instead of setting yourself up for yet another failure that adds even more pounds onto your frame, continuing to suffer from a lack of energy and possibly even poor health – *make a commitment to change the way you eat and your relationship with food* – starting right now!

Chapter Two

Strategy for Success

Finding a strategy for success when it comes to changing your eating habits can be a daunting process; but, the information that follows can help tremendously.

More than anything people just want to be healthy and to feel good about themselves. For those who want to lose weight – they just want to permanently lose those extra pounds they have been carrying around for months (or years).

So – what to do? Maybe it's time to take a different approach, embrace a new strategy that will help you succeed:

> ***Commit to changing your way of eating to one that will last a lifetime, instead of looking for a quick fix.***

Let's look at some habits that you must break to transform your current way of eating to a much healthier one.

Eliminate Time Markers

Deep down, healthy lifelong habits are what you really want. So, the first step is to forget about time parameters. Don't even think about starting another one of those highly-publicized diets that make ridiculous promises. Just focus on being a healthier person starting today – PERIOD!

When you remove the time pressure and focus on health, you open up a whole new world of possibilities.

In the beginning, you may not feel comfortable without time markers, because that is the way you have always done it – and that is the way the "experts" have told you to do it. BUT, remember you are going to do it differently this time!

It is okay to have goals . . . but . . . get rid of the end dates, PLEASE! The goal **to be healthy** is the only goal that matters.

No time markers for any reason – even if losing weight is part of your goal. ***Acknowledge and accept that accomplishing your goal will take as long as it takes***!

When you accept that fact without reservations, you have taken the first giant leap toward success.

What really matters is that you become healthier and begin to feel better – and, eventually, ***happy with the way you look.***

Change Your Focus

Developing a new way of eating must not focus on losing weight and body size. You must focus on choosing foods and eating habits that will effectively fuel your body for all its needs.

It should focus on eating nutrient-rich food that will help you reach a healthy weight for your personal height and body structure – not some societal image created by the media.

It should be on creating a mindset of self-care and protecting your health. Stop worrying about what others think about you.

When you change your eating patterns in the right way and for the right reasons, you will not only lose weight (if that is your goal); the changes can also help clear up your skin, increase healthy heart function, give you more energy, help you get pregnant (if that is a goal), build and sustain healthy brain function, decrease your risk of disease, etc.

You should not be looking for a new *diet*. That word can lead you astray because of its negative connotation – meaning a way of eating that is limiting, difficult to maintain, and something to dread.

You should be looking for a new *"way of eating."* A way of fueling your body to ensure physical peak performance, an efficiently functioning mind, and disease free (HEALTHY)!

Selecting and implementing a healthy "way of eating" can be challenging – especially if you have developed poor eating habits over a long period of time.

A recent FORBES article quoted Margaret Mead as saying, *"It is easier to change a man's religion than it is to change his diet."*

Which means you have your work cut out for you! ***The good news is that it can be done.***

Depending on your eating history and habits you have formed over many years, the complete evolution of the way <u>you</u> eat will take time. Be patient with yourself and the process (and it is a process) .

Chapter Three
Your Starting Point

An Introspective Evaluation

Most people live from day-to-day – even minute-to-minute – especially when it comes to food. They don't even think about their choices. They grab whatever is the easiest and the most appealing at the moment. Unfortunately, these are often empty-calorie foods that are filled with health-destroying additives.

For you to create a sustainable change in your life, it is critical to adopt a total mind and body wellness approach.

At birth, you were given the gift of life – a miraculous mind and body that cannot be replicated through technology. They have served you well and continue to function day-in and day-out, regardless of how you care for them.

It is time to acknowledge the importance and beauty of this gift and seriously consider how you want to care for it through your remaining years.

The first step is to take a <u>completely honest look at yourself</u> from head to toe, inside and out – physically, mentally, and emotionally.

Take the time to analyze your current mindset and the choices you make about the way you eat, plus the state of your physical body, and what you need to do to live and enjoy a healthier life. (Yes, that may include weight loss.)

Keep in mind, that how you feed and care for your body may be the only aspect of your life over which you have complete control – so, use that control wisely because it impacts every aspect of your life.

Ask and honestly answer all the hard questions. What do you really want out of life? Do you want a healthy, fit body filled with energy? Or, are you content with things the way they are?

Which of your daily behaviors contribute to good health, and should be sustained? What do you need to change in order to be physically healthy and to feel good mentality?

Do not fall into the trap of self-delusion, it will not serve you in this process.

The questions and answers should be written down (by hand or computer). DO NOT do this in your head. You need a record of your discoveries about your eating habits. You can find a form: ***Introspective Evaluation*** – in the Addendum.

This type of introspection may be difficult at first. But, once it is complete and you have clearly defined the type of life you want to live, you will feel more powerful, more clearly focused, and freer than you have been in the past. Making good choices as you move forward will be much easier than you ever thought possible.

It would be a mistake to skip this step because you are excited and ready to charge ahead with your new "lifestyle plan." Avoid tricking yourself into a false sense of security - thinking "I've got this" when in reality, you may not "have it."

It is critical to get real with yourself and honestly look at your current lifestyle including eating habits and physical behaviors (or lack thereof), and your emotional/mental attitudes about food over the years – especially the last three to five years.

It is also important to take into consideration any specific health issues you have, which can significantly impact your dietary needs.

This exercise will become the baseline from which all future steps will be taken. Don't go any further until you have answered the first set of questions in the *Introspective Evaluation*.

Chapter Four

Your Current Eating Habits

Hopefully, you completed the first part of the *Introspective Evaluation* in the Addendum, which will be your baseline or the starting point of your new lifestyle.

The next step is to complete a thorough examination of your current eating habits. In order to develop a healthy eating plan for moving forward, you must fully understand and acknowledge the truth about how you have been eating up to this point in time.

With that information, you will be able to identify the troublesome eating habits you need to change and the good eating habits you can continue and still stay healthy. This study must be done in three steps and it is as simple as A, B, C.

A. Keep a Record

The first step is to record everything you eat and drink for one week. This may be a pain in the "you-know-what" but it is important.

This is not about judgment or changing how you eat at this point – it is about collecting information to use later. Don't think about the process too much. Just eat as you always do and keep a record

Consistency and *honesty* are the critical factors required in keeping a useful food record. Unless you are willing to incorporate both of those into your record keeping, you will be wasting your time.

How you keep your records is unimportant – do what works for you. Use your computer, a mobile app on your phone, or even good old-fashioned pen and paper.

There is a **_FOOD DIARY_** that is accessible online and easy to use. When you register, it asks for some basic information and computes the number of calories you should be eating to lose weight. I don't recommend trying to lose more than one to two lbs. per week.

This program is a good choice if you will be keeping your record on a computer. You can get a free trial for seven days (perfect for this exercise). Then, if you want to continue, there is a small monthly fee.

I use apps on my Smart Phone, (a good choice if you have one). Two free apps that work well for tracking your food intake are **_Lose-it_** and **_My Plate._** They are very easy to use once you get used to them.

Each app has a large database, plus they track calories, your weight, and nutrients.

For this first week, your goal is to track what you are eating, the calorie intake, and your weight change (if any).

Before the convenience of apps, I <u>would not</u> have recommended recording what you eat for more than a couple of days, but now it is so easy that you will probably want to complete the full seven days.

If you do not have a Smart Phone, the next easiest choice is a computer, if that is not available. Pencil and paper will also work, it's just a little more labor intensive.

Record the food and amount as soon as you eat something. Try to keep the food intake in four groups: Breakfast, Lunch, Dinner, All Snacks.

Pay attention to the times of day that you eat – generally speaking. If you don't eat breakfast, that should be noted; and don't forget late night snacks.

The key factor is that you are diligent and completely honest about recording everything you eat each day.

Don't forget the extra doughnut your colleague offered you, the three pieces of candy you grabbed from the receptionist's candy dish or the Frappuccino you had as a pick-me-up in the afternoon.

You will need to know the type of food, the brand (if applicable), and the amount (oz/grams/number).

If a food choice is not listed in the database of the app, you can either scan it or "create your own food." A reliable calorie count can usually be found on Google, or you can bookmark a website like ***WEB MD Food Calculator.***

Where, When, and How

Where, when and how you eat are important when tracking eating habits.

- **Where do you eat?** Do you stand, sit at a table, eat while driving or walking? Do you eat at your desk while you are working? Do you eat your meals standing up or in your car because it is faster?

- **What time of day do you eat?** Do you skip breakfast? Do you just drinking coffee until noon, then eat lunch? Maybe you eat breakfast and dinner but skip lunch. Do you eat a couple of snacks in the am and pm, then have dinner? Do you have bedtime snacks?

- **How do you eat?** Do you graze or feast? Do you starve and then binge? Do you enjoy food, savoring each bite, or do you eat rapidly just to get it done? Do you always eat alone, or do you eat with friends and/or family? Do you grab all available snacks and gobble them down? Do you skip meals because you don't have time and then eat a candy bar in two or three bites because you are starving?

A few examples:

For breakfast, did you sit down for a nice breakfast with your kids and spouse? Did you stand up at the kitchen counter as you ate a quick bowl of cereal before rushing out the door? Or, did you just grab a quick latte at Starbucks on your way to work?

What did you do for lunch? Grab a coke and candy bar from the machine? Run to the nearest McDonalds? Eat the last doughnut from morning treats? Or, did you take some time in the lunch room to quietly enjoy the healthy sandwich you brought from home?

What about dinner? Did you sit on the couch mindlessly eating a frozen dinner and half a bag of chips as you watched TV? OR . . . did you take time to sit at the table for a healthy, relaxing meal with your family, a friend, or even by yourself?

Don't forget snacks? Did you grab a small bag of nuts or a piece of fruit for your morning snack? Did you buy a croissant or Cheese Danish with your morning coffee? Did you eat a couple of donuts brought in by a fellow worker? Did you buy a Big Gulp and a candy bar for the PM or did you get your favorite Starbucks Frappuccino as an afternoon pick-me-up? How about bedtime? Did you enjoy a three or four Oreos with a big glass of milk?

Keep good notes on all of this, including the time of day for each meal/snack.

Complete a summary at the end of each day. Everything will be fresh in your mind and you will be able to complete it quickly.

How you were feeling when you were eating? Were you stressed and anxious when you were eating a pint of ice cream last night? Were you rewarding yourself for a good day at work as you munched on a chocolate-filled croissant from the neighborhood bakery?

Why do you eat most of the time? Is it because you are hungry and your body needs refueling, or do you eat when you are upset, angry, sad, or lonely because it makes you feel better? Good records can help you identify triggers for mindless (and emotional) eating.

Were you consciously eating – or were you just eating? If you are not sure, make your best guess. Conscious, mindful eating may be a new concept for you; so, do the best you can in making that determination.

With the help of the information in this book, you will become more fully aware of what you are eating and why you are eating – both of which contribute to mindful eating.

Your new plan will focus on nutritional values, making good choices and ***what you do eat***, rather than what ***you cannot eat.***

Two additional things to track – for informational purposes only (both can be noted on the app you use):
1. Weigh yourself at the beginning of each week.
2. Keep track of the amount of water you drink each day.

B. Organize the Information

Once the seven days of record-keeping are complete you will have a lot of information; but, unless you organize it, study it carefully and learn the lessons that can be found there, it has no value.

Use the information to create a big picture of your current eating habits. Examine the picture carefully to glean the nuggets that will help you develop your new way of eating. Pay close attention to the following:

Categories of Food – Nutrients Are the Foundation

All the foods included in your seven-day record should fall into one of the following 10 categories.

Some of your food choices are rich in nutrients that are necessary for good health and should be included in your new way of eating (categories #1-5), others are empty calories (little or no nutrient value) and should be eliminated completely or eaten rarely, in small quantities (categories #6-10).

You also want to watch the carbs (#4) – healthy carbs are generally fine; but, go easy with the bad carbs. Be sure to get an adequate amount of protein and fiber. You can eat all the fruits and veggies that you want.

1. **PROTEIN (PRO)** – Building-block of the body; necessary for growth, good health, and body maintenance. *Foods high in protein are usually also high in calories.*
    - Eggs, beef, fish/shellfish, chicken, pork (including bacon, sausage, ham), lentils, beans, nuts, and some grains, i.e. quinoa.

    Be sure to eat an adequate amount of protein every day. As a general guideline, the DRI (Dietary Reference Intake) is 0.36 grams per pound of body weight. For a more accurate number for your own protein needs, use <u>Calculator.net.</u>

2. **DAIRY (D)** –Another good source of **protein**.
    - Milk, cottage cheese, all varieties of cheese, yogurt.

3. **FRUITS & VEGETABLES (F&V)** – Best source of **vitamins**. Also provides **fiber** and **minerals**. *You can eat unlimited amounts of vegetables and a generous amount of fruits every day – some have a higher calorie count than others.*

4. **CARBOHYDRATES (H-CARBS & B-CARBS)** – Provide necessary fuel for critical processes in your body – especially the central nervous system and brain; they also lower your risk for disease. *It is never a good idea to stop eating healthy carbs.*
    - *Healthy Carbs (eat)* – whole grains such as whole-wheat flour, quinoa, oatmeal; popcorn; nuts and seeds; beans and lentils; and fiber-rich fruits and vegetables such as: all berries, bananas, apples, pears, avocado, carrots, broccoli, artichokes, kale, sweet potatoes, and beets.
    - *Bad Carbs (avoid)* – All processed and refined foods such as white flour, rice, pasta, bread, crackers, cereal, and refined sugars like table sugar and high-fructose corn syrup. They are empty-calorie foods with no nutrient value and filled with additives.

5. **FATS (FAT)** – Necessary for vitamin and mineral absorption, blood clotting, building cells, and muscle movement. They act as an anti-inflammatory, help balance your blood sugar, improve brain function, and lower risk of arthritis, and Alzheimer's Disease.
    - *Healthy Fats (unsaturated)* – These can be found in nuts, seeds, avocados, and vegetable oils (olive, avocado, and flaxseed).
    - Healthy fats are high in calories – your intake should be less than 10% of your daily calories.
    - *Unhealthy Fats (trans-fats – AVOID Completely)*

6. **SUGAR AND SUGAR PRODUCTS (SGR)** – (AVOID) Empty-calories, refining process essentially removes all nutrients.
    - Most sweets, ice cream, candy, doughnuts, cookies, cake, pie, desserts. Anything made with white flour, processed sugar, added sugars of any kind, and high fructose corn syrup, etc.

7. **FAST FOODS (FF)** – (AVOID) - or indulge RARELY and choose carefully from the menu.

- McDonald's, Jack-in-Box, Wendy's, Canes, Sonic, Chick-Fil-A, In-and-Out, Taco Bell, White Castle, and any other establishment that you frequent.

8. **JUNK FOODS (JUNK)** – (AVOID) – unless you make them yourself from scratch, and then in limited quantities.
   - Generally, snack foods made of white flour, added sugars, and high sodium content such as Pop-Tarts, chips, crackers, pretzels, Cheetos, Packaged Fruit Pies, Snack Cakes, Donuts, Chocolate Candy Bars, etc.

9. **FLAVORED BEVERAGES (DRNK)** – (AVOID or limited amounts). Sugary drinks and energy drinks (high caffeine content) should be avoided completely. An occasional cup of coffee or herbal tea is acceptable; just don't fall into the habit of drinking many cups of fully caffeinated coffee every day.
   - Sodas, coffee (including cream/sugar), tea, energy drinks, hot chocolate, specialty beverages like lattes and Frappuccino, etc.

10. **PREPACKAGED/PROCESSED FOODS (PPP) – (AVOID COMPLETELY)** – There are loaded with poison additives and added sugars. Don't eat them. More and more studies are finding that consumption of heavily processed foods contributes to heart disease and early death.

Three additional components of eating well are:

WATER – *Keep your body hydrated.*
You can go for weeks without food, but no more than a few days without water. Every system in your body needs it. If you drink five or six 12-ounce bottles of water a day, you should be fine. But, water requirements can vary depending on your age, body size, air

temperature, climate conditions, physical activity, state of health, and types of food you eat.

Also – listen to your body, if you are thirsty – DRINK water!

The best way to tell if you are getting enough water is to check the frequency and color of your urine – it should be very pale yellow or nearly clear. If you do not urinate frequently and the color of your urine is dark yellow, you need more water.

FIBER – This nutrient is *often overlooked, but critical*, in order to maintain a healthy digestive tract and lower the risk of Type 2 Diabetes and colon cancer. It also helps with weight loss (helps you feel full), lowers blood sugar and cuts cholesterol levels.

Make every effort to get <u>at least</u> 38 grams daily (for men) and 28 grams daily (for women). Most people do not get enough!

- Fiber can be found in all types of fresh whole berries; dried fruits; fresh whole pears, apples, grapes with peeling; vegetables such as: corn, sweet potatoes, broccoli, Brussels sprouts, and zucchini; whole grain breads, cereals, and pasta; legumes, seeds, all nuts (especially almonds), and all types of beans.

Insert fiber into your diet slowly. It is not wise to go from very little fiber to a lot all at once. Add one or two servings a day. For example – have an apple or a handful of nuts for your afternoon snack instead of chips and a coke or add oatmeal to your smoothie.

Once you have built-up your intake to a healthy level, be sure to drink enough water (64 oz. a day), or you may find yourself constipated.

MINERALS - These are necessary for regulating metabolism, adequate hydration, and building strong bones and teeth. They also help maintain healthy blood pressure, muscle function, build healthy blood cells, and boost the immune system. If you *eat a well-balanced diet with plenty of*

fresh fruits and vegetables, in most cases you will get all the minerals you need.

Creating Your Big Picture

Using Excel (if available), create a chart like the one below to help you analyze your current eating patterns. There is also ***a form*** you can copy and use in the ***Introspective Evaluation***.

The good thing about using Excel is that you can sort by meals, by food type, category, nutrients, calories, etc. This will give you even more useful information.

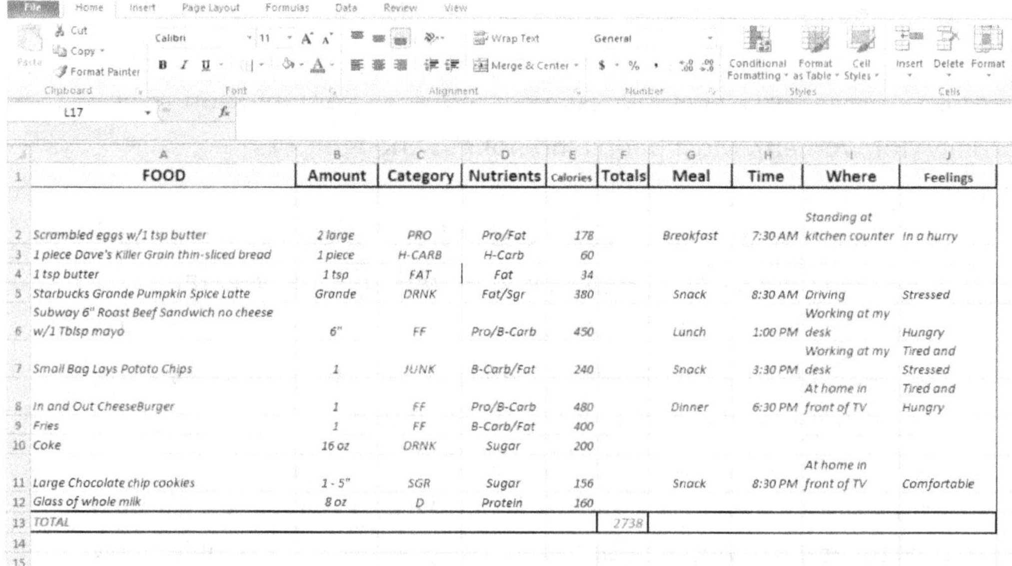

FOOD	Amount	Category	Nutrients	Calories	Totals	Meal	Time	Where	Feelings
Scrambled eggs w/1 tsp butter	2 large	PRO	Pro/Fat	178		Breakfast	7:30 AM	Standing at kitchen counter	In a hurry
1 piece Dave's Killer Grain thin-sliced bread	1 piece	H-CARB	H-Carb	60					
1 tsp butter	1 tsp	FAT	Fat	34					
Starbucks Grande Pumpkin Spice Latte	Grande	DRNK	Fat/Sgr	380		Snack	8:30 AM	Driving	Stressed
Subway 6" Roast Beef Sandwich no cheese w/1 Tblsp mayo	6"	FF	Pro/B-Carb	450		Lunch	1:00 PM	Working at my desk	Hungry
Small Bag Lays Potato Chips	1	JUNK	B-Carb/Fat	240		Snack	3:30 PM	Working at my desk	Tired and Stressed
In and Out CheeseBurger	1	FF	Pro/B-Carb	480		Dinner	6:30 PM	At home in front of TV	Tired and Hungry
Fries	1	FF	B-Carb/Fat	400					
Coke	16 oz	DRNK	Sugar	200					
Large Chocolate chip cookies	1 - 5"	SGR	Sugar	156		Snack	8:30 PM	At home in front of TV	Comfortable
Glass of whole milk	8 oz	D	Protein	160					
TOTAL					2738				

Enter everything you eat, day-by-day, during the seven days of tracking. I recommend that you complete the chart at the end of each day. It will be much easier than trying to do all seven days at once.

Note that there are several columns:
1. Food (include the source or brand)
2. Size of serving (oz/number/serving size)
3. Category: (PRO, H-CARB, B-CARB, SGR, FF, JUNK, PPP, etc.)

4. Nutrients
5. Calories
6. Total of daily calories
7. Breakfast, Lunch, Dinner, or Snack
8. Time of day you ate the meal/snack
9. What were you doing? (Sitting, standing, driving, etc.)
10. How were you feeling?

Please note the last question – ***How were you feeling?***
(Sad, hungry, happy, angry, tired, upset, stressed out, etc.) Feelings are a critical factor in your life for two reasons:

1. How you are feeling day-to-day is a strong indicator of how effectively your body is functioning – in other words, your overall well-being.
2. If you are eating because you are hungry, that's good. If you are eating to numb your emotions, that is not good.

Because of seriously unhealthy eating habits, there is an obesity epidemic in the United States.

Statistics show that 33.8% of adults are obese and approximately 17% of children and adolescents, ages 2 to 19, are obese.

Since dietary habits established in childhood usually carry over into adulthood, eating well and developing a healthy lifestyle is not only important for your own health, it is important for your children. Leading by example in the way you eat and helping them learn how to eat healthy at a young age will help them stay healthy throughout their lives

What You Eat Affects Your Mood

The food you choose to put into your body each day affects your health and how you feel today, tomorrow, and every day after that.

Many researchers believe that there is a link between depression and diet. They know for sure that certain foods will boost your mood: avocados, berries, tomatoes, leafy greens (spinach and kale), walnuts, seeds, and beans.

When you eat the right foods and combine it with regular physical activity you are more likely to reach and maintain a healthy weight and feel better mentally, as well.

C. Analyze the Information

The week is over, your daily charts are complete; so, the last step is to analyze the information you have collected This will help you recognize long-standing good habits, as well as bad habits that are sabotaging your efforts to be healthy (and lose weight, if that is your goal).

Lessons Learned

It is time to look at the results and summarize lessons learned. The list below can help you with the summary. Be sure to include any additional insights you gathered through the process that may not be included in the list.

1. Make two lists of your food choices:
   1) *Eat in Abundance*
   2) *Eat Occasionally or Not-at-all.*
2. How did your food choices either help you or hurt you?
3. What were your daily calorie intake and the average for the week?
4. Was there any weight variation (gain or loss)?
5. How did you feel physically throughout the week?
6. How did you feel mentally and emotionally throughout the week?
7. How was your energy? Did it vary at all?
8. Do you have any health conditions or concerns that improved or worsened?

The "Eat in Abundance" food list should be a list of nutritious foods that you enjoy and will sustain a healthy body. A list of these questions has been included in the ***Introspective Evaluation***.

When you provide your body with nutritious, healthy foods, it will have everything it needs to grow, develop, and age well.

You will be able to reach and maintain healthy body weight for your height and physical structure; you will be reducing the risk of chronic disease and will be able to look forward to good health and overall well-being for many years to come.

The key elements you are looking for are essential nutrients for building and sustaining good health: vitamins, protein, good carbohydrates, healthy fats, fiber, and plenty of water.

That doesn't mean you have to give up completely and forever the foods on the second list "Eat Occasionally or Not-at-all." Just don't eat them every day or in large quantities. They should be an occasional indulgence, nothing more.

As you analyze the information, stay out of judgment mode. At this point, you are creating a baseline from which you can plan and implement more effective eating patterns.

It would be smart to do additional research on your own regarding ways to eat healthily. It will give you valuable information to use as you develop your new way of eating.

A good place to start is an excellent article titled: _The 11 Most Nutrient-Dense Foods on the Planet._ You will probably be surprised by some, delighted by some, and maybe not so excited by some; but consider all of them carefully. Each one is a great choice as you will see when you read the article.

Two other articles that can be useful are: *Changing Your Diet: Choosing Nutrient-Rich Foods* and *Tips for Choosing a Nutrient-Rich Diet*.

As you study the articles, be sure to take good notes.
After you have completed the entire process of record keeping, organizing the information, analyzing and noting lessons learned, you will be ready to move on to the next chapter.

Chapter Five

Calories and Portion Control

In addition to choosing nutrient-rich foods, there are two more components to understand and factor-in when you are planning a healthy diet: calories and portion control.

Calories Are Important

Just the word "calories" make some people cringe; but, please stay with me on this.

The human body needs energy for organs to function normally and to keep you alive. The foods you eat and drink provide energy that fuels every movement your body makes from breathing to running.

The amount of energy in all foods is measured in calories. There are a few simple facts to remember about calories when planning a healthy diet:

- When you eat and drink more energy (calories) than the body needs, the excess calories are stored as fat. If you eat excess calories over time, you will probably gain weight.
- To lose weight, you need to use more energy (calories) than you consume over time.
- The number of calories needed vary with the individual and are determined by gender, height, current weight, body structure, general health, metabolism, and activity.
- The number of calories burned by a certain physical activity will vary depending on a range of factors, including physical size and age.
- A vigorous activity, burns more calories, e.g. a brisk, fast walk will burn more calories than a casual stroll.

How Many Calories Does Your Body Need?

Wouldn't it be lovely if all your favorite foods like wine and chocolate had no calories and you could have unlimited amounts of both and still maintain a healthy weight? Unfortunately, that is not the case. In fact, everything you eat or drink has calories – and they add up quickly.

In today's world, you can easily eat enough calories in one takeout meal that would meet your daily intake requirement. With office treats, fast-food chains everywhere, and unlimited tempting TV ads, it can be difficult to keep the calorie count under control.

But, if you know how many calories your body needs, and you have a good understanding of how many calories you have been eating daily, you will have taken the first step toward reaching and sustaining a healthy weight.

The FDA has chosen 2,000 calories to put on food labels as a rough average needed for daily intake. It is NOT a recommendation. The right number for you may be 2,000 calories – but, maybe not.

The number of calories **you need** depends on your age, height, current weight, metabolism, gender, physical health, and **activity level**. (Be careful with the last one. Most people overestimate how active they are. See **_Chapter Eight.)_**

Find out how many calories per day you need with this **_Calculator from Healthline or Calculator.net._** Either one will give you the numbers you need to maintain your weight, to lose weight and to lose weight fast – very useful information.

Factor-in what you know about your body. According to Calculator.net, I can lose weight at 1,500/day. I know from experience that I cannot. I must eat 1,200/day (or less) to lose weight.

Considering the results of the calculator and personal knowledge of your body, what are the correct numbers for you to maintain weight, to lose weight, and to lose weight fast? Enter those numbers on your *Introspective Evaluation.*

Once you understand how many calories your body needs and compare it with the number of calories you have been eating, you will have solid information that will guide you in making lasting changes.

Doing the math can help you be more mindful not only about what you eat but how much you eat. Always choose foods based on the nutrients they provide and the calorie count, which can be managed by portion control.

Calories in Food

Being aware of your daily calorie intake is an important part of the process. Using an app to track your calories is the easiest way to do that. When you get in the habit of entering the foods as soon as you eat, it quickly becomes a habit.

Everyone eats the same foods over-and-over again, so it doesn't take long before the foods you eat repeatedly are at the top of your meal lists in the app.

Tracking calories will help you identify patterns and habits that are holding you back and the source of excess calories.

The average American eats 3600 calories a day, which is far above the recommendation for the average person – man or woman. *(Be sure you enter your average daily intake of calories from the 7-day tracking exercise.)*

One of the main contributors to this problem is that people eat over-sized portions of high-calorie foods with limited nutrient value.

Most of these foods come from fast-food establishments, processed packaged foods and snacks, extra-large sodas, energy drinks, high-sugar content coffee drinks and all the other "convenience" foods that Americans love. Not only are they high-calorie and lacking in nutrients, but they are also filled with additives that poison your body.

Knowing how many calories you are consuming each day is vital. The calorie counting apps we have discussed will make calorie counting for your daily intake easy.

Without that information, you can overeat without realizing it. Once you understand nutrients, calories, and portion control, it will be much easier to reach a healthy weight and maintain it long-term.

It is also important to learn how to read labels and find the calorie count on all packaged goods. Be sure to check the serving size – sometimes it is ½ or ¼ of the package. If you are not careful, you may be eating many more calories than you think you are.

When you have the correct serving size and calorie count, you can quickly assess if a food fits into your daily eating plan.

You will find that many restaurants include calorie information on their menus (fast-food establishments do it too). If you pay attention, this information can help you make better choices when eating out; but, pay attention.

They often list a range of calories: 390 – 850. The lowest number is often a very plain serving without any sauces or trimmings (like cheese). Don't assume that what you are ordering contains the lowest number. If you order something with everything on it, you will probably be eating the highest number.

Portion Control Is Critical

It is a well-known fact that **Americans overeat!** In fact, Americans top the list as the biggest eaters in the world.

We serve extra-large portions on over-sized plates in our homes and buy the "supersize" of everything when we are out. The result is too much food and too many calories.

When you add the two problems together: large portions and high-calorie intake for almost every meal - every day of the year, people will be overweight and move quickly toward obesity.

There is no "one-size-fits-all" when it comes to recommended servings of any food. Portion recommendations vary with age, weight, height, gender, activity levels, health issues, and if you are pregnant or breastfeeding.

It is important to understand the correct portion size to properly fuel **your** body and to keep you fit and healthy at the same time.

Practice Portion Control

This may sound easier than it is because of long-established eating habits that can be difficult to change; plus, the food manufacturers purposefully mislead us with labeling practices.

Packaged foods typically contain more than one serving size (written in fine print), but you think it is only one and eat the whole thing. It is important to check the "number of servings" listed on food labels and eat only one serving, which is usually half the package.

For fresh foods (meat, vegetables, potatoes, etc.) there are some basic rules to help keep your portions in check.
- A good serving of meat is the size of a deck of cards.

- A serving of fruits and vegetables should be about the size of an average fist.
- A serving of starchy foods – like potatoes, rice, and corn – should be the size of a computer mouse (which is not very big).

See the ***Portion Guidelines*** in the Addendum for additional healthy portion sizes.

How Much Are You Currently Eating?

Check Your Portions
For the next few days, serve yourself as you normally would. Don't think about it and don't measure. Once your plate is full, measure the food so that you can see how much you take.

Don't Hide the Truth from Yourself
You will probably be surprised at how much you have been eating. You may think you have been eating ½ cup of mashed potatoes, and when you measure the serving you realize it is closer to 2½ cups.

Check the Size of Your Dinner Plates
Are they small, medium, large, oversized? The average American dinner plate is 11 to 12 inches across. Only a few decades ago they were 7 to 9 inches. Most restaurants use 13-inch plates.

Since 1960 the overall surface area of an average dinner plate has increased by 36%. As plate sizes grew, so did the portions, which has fooled all of us into thinking that we are eating normal amounts of food.

Research has shown that if you switch from a 12-inch plate to a 10-inch plate, you will eat 22% less food – an 8 or 9-inch plate is even better. It is interesting to note that when you eat from a smaller plate, you still feel full and satisfied even though you are eating less.

Invest in Smaller Dinner Plates

The 8-inch plate is recommended. Do not go above 9-inches. The smaller plates are usually called lunch plates. If the description reads "dinner plate," be careful. Be sure to check the size before you buy or you may end up with additional, large dinner plates.

The smaller plates are available online (Wayfair and Amazon), or at your local Target or Walmart.

A Quick Evaluation

Think for a moment about the last few meals you have eaten and answer the following questions:

What size plate do you normally use? Do you have the large dinner plates in your home that are used regularly? Or, do you have the smaller "lunch" plates?

How did you fill your plate?
Was it stacked to overflowing, or was there actually white space showing? This is particularly a problem with the bigger plates.

Which foods took up most of the room on your plate?
Meat or fatty foods like Mac & Cheese? Or, mashed potatoes smothered with butter or gravy? Were there any vegetables or whole grains? If either of those were on your plate, what was the portion size compared to the other foods?

Be honest in this evaluation. It is important to see how your typical plate looks against the health and wellness plates you plan to prepare in the future for your new way of eating.

Identify Your Eating Pattern

How Often Do You Eat?

Over the past several years, the trending recommendation has been to eat smaller amounts (mini-meals) 5-6 times a day, rather than the traditional three full meals a day – breakfast, lunch, and dinner, plus healthy snacks, if needed.

Another mandate that you have heard is: Always eat breakfast, which you may or may not do.

You are the only one who can decide what works best for you – and make a choice of how you are going to eat in the future.

Mini-Meals (Eat 5-6 times a day)

People who choose this eating pattern are sometimes called **grazers.** They seem to eat all the time – from their first cup of coffee to their late-night snack. They eat small portions of food – here and there – all day long rather than eating full-sized meals.

Strategically, choosing to eat six small nutritious meals a day rather than three large ones can be effective. But, if you are stress eating, or snacking on the wrong kinds of food all day – propping your body up with a non-stop sugar rush – rather than choosing healthy foods, you are endangering your health.

Some negatives to consider:
- You think about food all the time.
- You eat out-of-habit, rather than because you are hungry.
- You never feel hungry because you lose contact with your body's hunger cues.
- It may or may not boost your metabolism (not yet proven).

- Your body adjusts to a constant supply of energy, which makes it less likely to burn fat for energy.
- Your body is forced to constantly restart the digestive system, which can impair digestion.

Other factors to consider:
- Some people do not have huge appetites and can only eat a small amount at a time. This is often true with seniors.
- Professional responsibilities or the daily routine (i.e. being a mom) makes sitting down to full meals challenging.
- Health issues such as diabetes or hypoglycemia require individuals to eat more often.

On the other hand, eating frequently can be a problem for those who tend to overeat for any reason:
- Problems with portion control – bigger is always better.
- Stimulus-bound eating (sight of certain foods, prompts eating it) – i.e., chips, pretzels, chocolate.
- If given the chance to eat, they eat – any type of food, healthy or not. Free snacks in the company break room cannot be passed up.
- All or nothing eater – a small snack turns into a bigger one - instead of enjoying a few nuts, they just keep eating and eating.

Traditional Three Meals a Day

According to Ayurveda, three meals a day is ideal for healthy digestion and effective assimilation of nutrients.

People who eat three meals a day generally eat to fuel their body. Many also simply enjoy sitting down, relaxing, and savoring the food. This group is sometimes called ***feasters.***

They typically start with a hearty breakfast, work all morning, stop for more fuel at lunch, and again at dinnertime when the day is done.

They *do not typically* snack between meals unless their hunger cues are so persistent they cannot ignore them. This is the more traditional approach to eating and is preferred by those who enjoy feeling full and re-energized after a good meal.

Three meals a day with hours in-between allow people to stay in tune with natural hunger cues which the body sends out when it is functioning properly. You may become cranky, have difficulty concentrating, feel tired, have a slight headache, or a growling stomach.

Hunger comes on slowly and it is physical. When you eat all the time, it can be hard to tune-into these cues.

Both Patterns Work

You can feel good and lose weight with both styles. The key to success is two-pronged: 1) Choose healthy foods that satisfy your hunger. 2) DO NOT fill-up on empty-calories or stuff yourself every time you sit down to eat.

In making the transition to healthier foods, it may be easier to continue with your preferred schedule (graze or feast) in the beginning.

Once you become comfortable with healthier foods and feel confident about your new diet (lifestyle), you may begin to realize that switching eating patterns (grazer to feaster – or – feaster to grazer) may be a better choice for you.

Final Consideration – to Eat or Not Eat Breakfast

You have probably heard that breakfast is important because it jump-starts your metabolism for the day.

There are also studies that show people who skip breakfast are more likely to be obese. This conclusion may be tied to the fact that breakfast-skippers are more typically less health-conscious overall.

There is no solid evidence that supports the habit of eating breakfast jump-starts your metabolism or helps you lose weight.

Personally, I believe breakfast is important. You should eat something – a piece of fruit, whole-grain toast with peanut butter, or a glass of freshly squeezed juice. Keep in mind that you have been fasting for 10-12 hours and the body needs nutrients for energy and water for hydration.

There are also studies that show:
- The body's blood sugar control is better in the morning; so, eating breakfast results in lower average daily blood sugar levels.
- People with Type 2 Diabetes who don't eat until lunch will have increased blood sugar levels after eating lunch and dinner.

Conclusion, regarding breakfast, is that anyone struggling with blood sugar levels (hypoglycemia or Type 2 Diabetes) should eat a healthy breakfast.

For all other adults (not children), if you are not hungry in the morning, it is not a disaster if you skip breakfast; but . . . make sure that you drink water to stay hydrated and eat healthy foods for the rest of the day. On the other hand, . . . if your body says, "I'm hungry" – don't ignore the signals – stop and EAT (healthy food, of course).

Summary

Everyone is different when it comes to eating patterns. Ask yourself, *"What are my current eating habits and are they working for me? Is a change required?"*

Complete the questions on the Evaluation in connection with this section.

It has not been scientifically proven that one eating pattern is better than the other. Eating more often does not increase calories burned, help with weight loss, or improve blood sugar control. In fact, if anything, eating fewer meals seems to be healthier.

You must decide what works for you and will be the most helpful in reaching your goals. Regardless of the choice you make, use the following as your mantra:

When you are hungry, EAT!

When you are full, STOP!

When you are thirsty, DRINK water!

Chapter Six

State of Your Health

Your current state of health should be factored into your planning. The following is for informational purposes only and is not meant to be accepted as medical advice – that must come from a licensed health-care professional.

Food choices and types of diets are endless; but, selecting a way of eating that nourishes the whole body is more likely to offer long-term success because you will be improving your health and feeling better as you change your eating habits.

If you keep a wholistic mindset, you will choose a way of eating that addresses all the needs of your body, including health issues of any kind.

Low Energy

Practically everyone who tries to lose weight must deal with the *loss of energy* at some point – often in the beginning.

Your body has adjusted to your regular eating patterns and when those are changed significantly – it must adjust again. This often results in some energy fluctuations throughout the day.

Energy fluctuations can also be the result of poor dietary habits, lack of sleep, or exercise patterns. If you suffer fluctuations that are severe and frequent, such as bouts of energy loss so great that it is difficult to put one foot in front of the other, consult your physician.

If there is no underlying health issue; but, you struggle with the mid-afternoon energy drop each day, be sure you eat foods that will boost and sustain energy levels from morning to night.

If you know that energy fluctuations are one of your challenges, the "mini-meals 5-6 times a day" may be a better choice for you. It may be more effective in providing the fuel your body needs to run smoothly and function well until day's end.

Be sure that you choose stamina-building, energy-boosting foods that are loaded with high fiber foods and complex carbohydrates. *A low-carbohydrate diet would probably not be a good choice.*

Vagaries of Age

The foods you eat affect every part of your body – including all your organs (from the skin to the heart). The effect can be positive or negative. The foods you have eaten all your life have contributed to your aging process – sometimes negatively.

 If you consume a lot of red meat and other fatty foods, not only will your skin age faster, you will also experience internal cellular aging, as well.

All good anti-aging eating plans have one thing in common. They focus on eating fresh, healthy foods (as close to their natural state as possible) and can also offer a safe rate of weight loss.

Anti-aging foods include lots of fresh fruits and vegetables for the vitamins, minerals, and antioxidants to keep your eyesight in good condition and help prevent cancer; plenty of whole grains (which help blood vessels stay healthy); plus, fish and lean meats as the preferred protein for your meals. Fish is rich in Omega-3, which fights memory loss and helps maintain strong cognitive skills.

The *Mediterranean Diet* fills all those requirements. It is a good choice for those who want to look younger and live longer.

Cancer

Cancer is more prevalent today than it has ever been! True? Maybe – maybe not. Maybe we are simply more aware of cancer because of early detection tests.

Unfortunately, there are numerous studies which show the average American diet is primarily made up of sugary, fatty, processed foods filled with additives that cause disease rather than support the body's immune system in fighting it – especially cancer.

Fast foods and convenient, packaged, processed foods are huge temptations for busy people – especially working moms and overworked professionals.

Also, for single people, it is especially easy to fall into the habit of grabbing whatever is quick and easy (and requires no work). Preparing healthy meals for one requires a serious commitment to healthy eating.

What the average person does not realize is that eating healthier is not difficult – it simply takes commitment and planning.

The long-term benefits to your body are well worth the effort. The primary focus of your eating plan should be to help protect your body from all diseases – especially cancer and other debilitating conditions like diabetes.

If you would feel more comfortable with an actual "Diet Plan" – consider the *Mediterranean Diet.* In all my research, this one seems to be the healthiest option for most people.

The American Journal of Clinical Nutrition published a story that showed the benefits of the *Mediterranean Diet* against the risk of getting breast cancer. The diet avoids saturated fats and processed foods filled with ingredients that harm the body. It is rich in antioxidants and fish containing Omega 3 – both important in the fight against cancer.

Diabetes

If you have been diagnosed with pre-diabetes or diabetes, stabilizing your blood sugar should be a priority to prevent full-blown diabetes or to get it under control in order to avoid long-term health problems that diabetes can cause. You should be under a doctor's care and guidance when it comes to your eating plan.

For Type 2 Diabetes, there are some good options if weight loss is your goal. According to several nutritionists, if you want a "Diet Plan" there are two you should consider (with approval from your doctor):

1. The *DASH Diet*. It is a plant-based plan that is rich in fruit, vegetables, nuts, and legumes. It also includes low-fat dairy, lean meat, fish, poultry, whole grains, and heart-healthy fats, such as: avocados, nuts, fish and olive oil.

2. The *Mediterranean Diet* is also recommended because of its emphasis on fresh seasonal foods and produce, fish, and a little wine. However, be careful with the carbs – 50% of the foods come from carbs (healthy ones), but still, proceed with caution. It may be wise to work with a dietician if this is your choice.

Heart Disease

Blood pressure can be a precursor to heart disease. Fortunately, there are diets that can help you control blood pressure problems. The *DASH Diet* (Dietary Approach to Stop Hypertension) is recommended by the National Institutes of Health for people with hypertension.

The key elements of any diet to control blood pressure are low-sodium meals made up of healthy foods like fruits and vegetables, low-fat dairy, lean meats, and no alcohol.

One way to begin is to create a daily meal plan that emphasizes vegetables, fruits, and whole grains. It should limit high-fat foods (such as red meat, cheese, and baked goods) and high-sodium foods (such as canned or processed foods).

If you have any type of heart condition, please, consult with your doctor before deciding on a new way of eating.

Chronic Inflammation

Lifestyle factors like stress and a lack of exercise can lead to problems with chronic inflammation. This happens when the immune system releases chemicals meant to combat injury and bacterial or virus infections, even when there are no foreign invaders to fight off. In other words, the immune system goes out of control.

Chronic low-grade inflammation can eventually cause serious problems – such as rheumatoid arthritis and a host of other health problems, including cancer and depression.

When you are suffering from inflammation (short- or long-term), you generally feel miserable. A well-thought-out eating plan can give your body some relief.

Foods that are high in sugar and saturated fats can trigger certain types of inflammation. If you have been struggling with any kind of inflammatory disease or have arthritis in your joints that seems to be getting worse, it would be wise to consider the types of food you are eating regularly. They may be triggering your flare ups.

To help alleviate the problem, you should start by eliminating all white sugar and white flour products as well as processed foods that are filled with additives.

Then, be sure to implement an anti-inflammatory eating plan designed to prevent or reduce low-grade chronic inflammation. It should include lots of fruits, vegetables, lean protein, nuts, seeds, and healthy fats.

One diet that is often recommended for people with chronic inflammation is the **Flexitarian (Flexible Vegetarian).** This was created by a dietitian, **_Dawn Jackson Blatner,_** to help people reap the benefits of being a vegetarian, but still enjoy animal products in moderation.

The Flexitarian Diet is unlike other diets because it has no clear-cut rules. It is more of a lifestyle than a diet, but it is based on the following principles:

- The foundation of the diet is mostly fruits, vegetables, legumes, and whole grains.
- Most protein will come from plants rather than animals, but some animal protein is allowed (this is where the flexible part comes in).
- Eat foods in the most natural form possible and avoid processed foods altogether.
- Avoid (or limit) added sugars and sweets.

Because the diet is truly flexible and focuses on what you can eat, rather than on what you cannot eat, the Flexitarian Diet is very popular among people who want to eat healthier. As you can see, it fits nicely into our purpose for this book.

Eating as a vegetarian – even part-time by incorporating vegetarian meals two or three times a week can make a difference in how you feel. Foods such as whole grains, baked fish, dark leafy greens, almonds, low-fat dairy, tomatoes, and beets are all good food choices for fighting inflammation.

Depression

Depression is the leading cause of disability in Americans ages 15 to 44. It impacts more than 16 million adults in the United States each year. Studies show that foods you eat or don't eat may affect how you feel.

In a recent paper, researchers analyzed the results of 41 studies on depression and food. They found eating a **_Mediterranean diet_** was linked to a 33 percent lower risk of depression.

We have already discussed the makeup of this diet and its emphasis on natural foods/produce, and fish. One of the main reasons it is effective for people suffering from depression according to Charles Conway, Ph.D. at Washington University in St. Louis, is because of the omega three fatty acids that come from fish. He states, "They are known to have pretty clear effects with depression."

It has also been found that a diet high in processed foods, sugar, and saturated fats increased the risk of depression. It is important that people struggling with this life-threatening condition should avoid all processed flour and sugar, plus all products made from them; also, hydrogenated oil, artificial sweeteners, heavy intake of caffeine, and high fructose corn syrup.

Some foods that have been shown to boost your mood are avocados, berries, tomatoes, leafy greens like kale and spinach, walnuts, seeds, and beans.

If you eat a regular diet of healthy foods, including the foods listed above; and, add a good routine of physical activity (which we will discuss further in **_Chapter Eight_**), you will be helping both your mind and body in their fight against depression.

Other Health Concerns

Allergies

If you have been diagnosed with a dangerous food allergy such as nuts or shellfish or if you suffer from celiac disease and require a gluten-free diet, you must be responsible and take care of yourself in those areas.

For all others, don't foolishly "jump on the bandwagon" just because something has become popular or is well-advertised. You may be putting yourself at risk.

A study published in The BMJ in 2017 concluded that a person who follows a gluten-free diet without having celiac disease has a higher risk of cardiovascular disease in the long term. This is because they will miss out on the heart-healthy benefits of whole grains.

Unless you have a doctor-confirmed health reason for not eating a specific food such as whole grains, you should NOT eliminate them from your diet.

There are no proven cures for seasonal allergies, but it is a sure thing that fruits and vegetables are full of nutrients that can keep you healthier. Some experts believe that they may also protect you from the sniffles, eye itching, and the aggravation of seasonal allergies.

Web M.D. recommends the following foods to fight seasonal allergies:

1. Onions, peppers, berries, and parsley contain a chemical that may reduce "histamine reactions." Histamines are part of the allergic response.
2. Kiwi, oranges, and other citrus fruits contain Vitamin C that cuts down on histamines.
3. Pineapple has an enzyme called bromelain that can reduce irritation in allergic diseases such as asthma.
4. Tuna, salmon, and mackerel contain Omega-3 fatty acids that help reduce inflammation.

5. Kefir, sauerkraut, and kimchi are good sources of probiotics that may help prevent and even treat seasonal allergies.
6. Local Honey – there are mixed opinions about local honey and allergies, but it is tasty and if it may help, why not eat it?

Indigestion

Fruits and vegetables are generally beneficial for all users – except people who struggle with indigestion. If you suffer from this, stay away from acidic foods that can worsen indigestion. Avoid citric- and tomato-based foods as well as caffeine, sodas, red meat, garlic, and spicy foods. You may only need to stop eating them in the evening hours.

If you are having serious digestive system problems or if there is even the possibility that you have a serious problem such as acid reflux, irritable bowel syndrome, ulcers, celiac disease, etc., please consult a physician as soon as possible.

Insomnia

According to the Alaska Sleep Education center, there are four main vitamins and minerals that can be found in food that aid in promoting sleep: tryptophan, magnesium, calcium, and B6.

The following foods contain some, or all, of the vitamins and minerals that promote sleep:
- Milk, yogurt, cheese
- Poultry and seafood
- Bananas, avocados, peaches
- Cashews, almonds, walnuts
- Green leafy vegetables

The reason those foods help with sleep is that they turn serotonin into melatonin. There are also a few foods that are excellent sources of **_naturally occurring melatonin_**
- Tart cherries, corn, asparagus, tomatoes, pomegranate, olives, grapes, broccoli, cucumber.

- Rice, barley, rolled oats.
- Nuts and Seeds (walnuts, peanuts, sunflower seeds).

Drinks that will help you sleep:
- Warm milk (regular or almond)
- Valerian, chamomile, passion fruit or peppermint tea
- Tart cherry juice

There are also foods/eating habits that can rob you of sleep:
- Caffeine
- Very dark chocolate
- Spicy foods
- Alcohol
- High-fat and high-protein foods
- Eating heavy meals before bedtime

If you want to leave insomnia behind, try doing it naturally through healthy foods and good eating habits before resorting to medication.

Skin Problems

Diets with lots of fish, especially salmon are good. Blueberries are great at correcting skin problems, too. However, avoid pineapple because it can cause flare-ups as can certain spices.

Stress

A poor diet can be extremely stressful on your body and put you at risk for many diseases and debilitating conditions. A healthy diet can be one of your best weapons for managing stress.

Web MD food recommendations to tame stress:

- **Complex carbs:** whole-grain bread, pasta, and breakfast cereal, including old-fashioned oatmeal. They help the body produce serotonin and stabilize blood sugar levels.

- **Foods rich in Vitamin C:** oranges (all citrus) and kiwi fruit. This vitamin curbs levels of stress hormones and strengthens the immune system.

- **Magnesium-rich foods**: green leafy vegetables and salmon top the list. A magnesium deficiency can trigger headaches and fatigue, which intensifies stress.

- **Omega-3 fatty acids:** salmon and tuna are excellent sources and should be eaten twice a week. These acids prevent surges of stress hormones and may help protect against heart disease, depression, and PMS.

- **Healthy fats from nuts:** pistachios, almonds, walnuts. A handful a day can help protect you against the effects of stress; plus, they may help lower your cholesterol, ease inflammation in your arteries, and make diabetes less likely. ***NOTE: Nuts are loaded with calories.***

  Almonds are also loaded with Vitamin E that bolsters the immune system and Vitamin B that will help you manage stress and bouts of depression.

- **Potassium-rich foods:** Avocados are at the top of the list, bananas come in second, but are also good. Potassium helps lower blood pressure, which often results in stress overload. Avocados are high in calories so eat in small portions.

- **Crunchy raw vegetables:** carrots and celery are high on the list. Not only are they filled with vitamins and minerals, but the simple act of munching on them helps alleviate stress because it can release a clenched jaw and ward off increased tension.

- **Warm milk at bedtime:** It has been long accepted that calcium eases anxiety, helps you relax and go to sleep.

Stress relief and management are critical to good health. If you struggle with stress overload, eating healthy is only part of the solution, you should also exercise at least four times a week. If needed, consider supplements that can also help. *(See Chapter Eleven)*

Smoking

This is a bad habit that can create health issues and should be broken as quickly as possible. According to Dr. Andy McEwen from the National Centre for Smoking Cessation and Training:

> *Smoking affects the body's ability to absorb a variety of vitamins and minerals including calcium and Vitamins C and D. Smoking also affects the body's circulation by causing blood vessels to narrow and become blocked because of an increased build-up of fatty deposits. Stopping smoking is an effective method of helping avoid deficiencies of vitamins.*

Not only can your diet curb your smoking, it can also help repair damage done to the body by smoking.

Unhealthy foods such as caffeinated drinks, alcoholic beverages, and meat products make smoking taste better while other foods, such as fruits/vegetables, non-caffeinated beverages, and dairy products, make a cigarette taste worse.

Summary

Never choose an eating plan based solely on how many pounds you can lose in the shortest amount of time. Focus on *looking good and feeling great for the rest of your life.*

You not only want to reach a healthy weight that fits your body structure, you also want longevity and good health. So . . . it is important to make your food choices based on the health benefits that match your body's needs.

Chapter Seven

Trim Down by Eating Healthy

If you are among the many who want and/or need to lose weight, the first instinct for most people is to look for a diet that will help them lose weight fast.

They jump on the newest, highly-publicized diet plan that will crank up their metabolism and burn more calories than they take in so that the weight falls off quickly. There is little or no consideration of the overall impact on their mental and physical health.

It is time to stop taking this approach!

Choose a Healthy Plan that You Can Manage

Long-term good health (not weight loss) should be your primary focus when choosing a plan to help you lose weight. A healthy diet cannot be centered on how much you weigh, depriving yourself of foods you love, or based on extreme eating philosophies.

If you have gone through the exercises in Chapters 3, 4, and 5, and are committed to healthy eating, you should be clear on what you want to accomplish over the long-term with your new healthy lifestyle. Those goals should guide you in choosing the best plan to help you lose weight.

You should also consider the following:

Your Daily Schedule and Obligations
What is required of you every day? If you are an extremely busy person (professionally or as a parent), it may be wise to choose a plan that includes pre-packaged food or foods that are easy to prepare ahead of time – such as **Jenny Craig** or **Nutrisystem.**

These "convenient" plans can be very useful – especially during the first month until you get into the rhythm of eating differently.

I do not recommend staying on this type of diet for very long – possibly a month to kick-start the weight loss and to learn portion control. The primary reasons for not continuing are the number of preservatives (additives) in the pre-packaged foods, the taste of the food gets very old, very fast – and they are expensive.

For those who have a little more time and flexibility, you may want to choose a meal plan where you can take advantage of the opportunity to prepare fresh foods for all meals. This is by far the best choice if you can manage it.

If that appeals to you, the **Mediterranean Diet** is an excellent plan to follow. The **U.S. News and World Report** ranked the Mediterranean diet as the best diet for 2019 because it's accessible, sustainable, and not restrictive. The focus is on plant-based foods, fruits, vegetables, olive oil, and fish.

Long-term studies have found that if you follow the Mediterranean diet correctly, you can reap the full benefits, such as reduced risk of developing cardiovascular disease, kidney disease, and breast cancer. It can also help improve cholesterol levels, assist in weight loss, and even extend your life.

There are several goods books available that can guide you through this way of eating. Check out the following article: _The 10 Best Mediterranean Diet Books (2019)._

The State of Your Health
If you are lucky enough to be healthy and without any serious health issues, you may want to choose a diet that lets you consume some of your favorite foods.

For example, if you are a big meat eater, it would be cruel to go straight vegan or vegetarian and be forced to give up meat entirely. Going meatless two or three nights a week makes sense for future health reasons, but there is no reason to jump to extremes that will only make you miserable.

The **Mediterranean** or **Flexitarian Diet** would be better choices. (See the article: The Flexitarian Diet: A Detailed Beginner's Guide.)

No matter which path you choose to follow – healthy eating is critical. Be sure you get the calories and nutrients your body needs. No matter how much weight you lose and how thin you become, if you end up hospitalized due to poor health issues that you chose to ignore for the thrill of dropping two or three dress (or pant) sizes, it is not worth it.

A Plan that Fits Your Budget

You may really love the idea of prepackaged meals like Jenny Craig or Nutrisystem, but they are pricey!

Eating natural fresh foods is usually a much better choice. Some people complain that fruits and vegetables are too costly. It is true some are expensive; but, there are plenty of affordable options.

Organic used to be hard to find and prohibitively costly. That is no longer the case. Most grocery stores have a complete organic produce section and it is often close in cost or only slightly higher than the regular produce.
-    Learn to shop sales, buy fruits that are in season, and stock up on produce that lasts longer – like apples and oranges.
-    Whole fruits and vegetables are more budget-friendly than pre-washed, chopped and pre-packaged fruit, veggies and salad makings. Convenience packaging can quickly put a hole in your budget.

Seven Tips for Buying Healthier Foods

For centuries, individuals and families were responsible for food production. They hunted, fished, raised cattle, chickens, and pigs, tended to large productive gardens, and had fruit trees and grapevines on their property. What was not produced at home was obtained through bartering with friends and neighbors.

Things have changed dramatically. People have moved into the cities and no longer have the land (or the desire) to "grow their own" food, which has separated us completely from the process of food production. We now rely on major corporations to decide which foods will be available to us – and in many cases – how they will be prepared.

Advanced technology has also been incorporated into the way food is farmed and produced. Most of the food eaten today comes from huge factory farms so massive that the contamination factor is a serious problem. The situation has hit crisis level and it is time to take control of the food you eat.

Being in control requires that you educate yourself about how food is grown and processed. Be knowledgeable about healthy available foods, pay attention when you shop, read labels, and avoid anything that contains harmful ingredients.

1.   *Buy grass-fed and pastured meats*
Factory farms mistreat their animals and feed them sub-standard food. When you consume an unhealthy animal, you are not providing adequate nutrition to your own body. Animals allowed to graze and eat a diet natural to them are leaner than their "fattened" counterparts, they have more omega-3 fatty acids, and they are more nutrient dense.

Search the Internet for local producers of grass-fed, natural beef and other safe meats (without hormones, antibiotics or GMOs). If you cannot find a local producer, look for one that will ship frozen cuts of meat.

2. *Buy pasture-raised eggs (if possible from a local farmer)*

The Sprouting Seed.com explains the reasons why pastured eggs are the healthiest, "The birds run free in the pasture and eat a natural diet that is made up of all kinds of seeds, green plants, insects and worms. Usually grain or laying mash supplements the diet. Hens are allowed access to pasture, but also have a pen to house them and protect them from predators. This is not only more humane for the chickens, but also produces much healthier eggs." (BTW – Cage Free is not the same thing.)

3. *Shop the farmer's market for local food*

Local grocery store chains are getting better about stocking organic fruits and vegetables, but the fact remains that their produce is often harvested weeks in advance and transported many miles to get to you. So, even though they are organic, the term "fresh" is questionable, which means that nutrient loss is a certainty – and significant.

Every big city that I have lived in, including New York City, has a farmer's market. As a rule, these markets offer fresh fruits and veggies that are picked the morning of the day you are buying. If you live in or near a rural area, you can possibly find local farmers to buy from directly. Either of these is a much better choice than the local grocery store.

If you have no idea where to start, use the Internet to check out the CSA (Community Support Agriculture) in your area. A CSA gives city dwellers the opportunity to enjoy quality, fresh produce grown locally by regional farmers.

If you become a member of a CSA you will purchase a "share" of vegetables from a regional farmer. The season typically runs from June until October with weekly or bi-weekly deliveries to a drop-off location in (or near) your neighborhood.

At the very least, take a drive this weekend and visit local farms in your area. You may be surprised at what you discover.

4. Grow your own or pick your own

Gardening may not be your thing. Some people feel intimidated by the thought of growing their own vegetables and fruit. There is absolutely no reason to feel that way. It is quite easy, especially if you start small.

Choose one or two items that your family enjoys and plant them in large pots or raised beds around the perimeter of your yard. You can either start them from seeds or buy starter plants from the local nursery. Two easy ones to grow are tomatoes and strawberries – both tasty, healthy additions to your diet, and relatively easy to grow.

If time, hectic schedules, and no space at all are factors that would prevent you from growing your own, you can often find local pick-your-own farms. These types of farms provide carrying containers and allow you to walk the rows and pick your own food. Many delicious choices are available: sweet corn, pumpkins, strawberries, blackberries, raspberries, squash, and beans.

Depending on the region in which you live, you may find pick-your-own orchards for apples, pears, apricots, plums, and peaches. When you get home, you can immediately enjoy the sweet freshness of the fruit, prepare frozen dishes for future delight, and even learn to bottle them for the winter months when the fruits are out-of-season.

If all else fails, buy the freshest organic offerings at your local grocery store. If you have a *Sprouts* or *Trader Joes* in your area, they typically offer a nice variety of reasonably fresh, organic produce at fair prices.

5. Do not buy processed foods

This includes all white flour and white sugar products. They have been stripped of nutrients and are nothing more than empty calories that hurt your body more than help it.

Processed foods are typically filled with preservatives/additives that are poisonous to your body and added sugars. Both put you at risk for serious health problems. The best way to avoid them is to buy foods as close to their natural state as possible – as described in numbers 1-4 above.

If you must buy packaged goods – learn to read labels carefully. Check the ingredients first. Look for high-fructose corn syrup, added sugars, preservatives, and words you don't recognize or cannot pronounce. If any of those are included, do not buy it.

A simple rule-of-thumb is: *If what you are buying contains more than five ingredients and includes a lot of unfamiliar, unpronounceable items, you should reconsider before buying.*

Frozen vegetables and fruits are fine if there is nothing but the fruit in the package! The quick-freeze process helps preserve nutrients and freshness, so they can be an excellent substitute for fresh produce.

Canned goods are also OK in a pinch. It is it best to buy low-sodium, if available. Again, check the label and be sure there is nothing except the fruit or vegetable, water, and a small amount of salt (if any).

6. *Buy bread from a local bakery*

If you check the label on most bread, you may be shocked at the list of ingredients. Bread from a local bakery is more likely to be made of the simple list of ingredients required for bread – you can ask them for an ingredient list if you would like.

When it comes to other grain products – always go for the whole-grain option. Do not take health claims on the box seriously. Read the label and verify that it is made with 100% whole grains – not a combination of whole grains and refined grains which is unfortunately how a lot of so-called "whole grain" products are made.

7. *Do not buy foods that contain added sugars by any name*
Sugar in foods comes in a plethora of forms. You must be a detective in order to avoid it when you are grocery shopping. Below is a list of sugars without the name "sugar."

- Barley malt syrup
- Corn sweetener
- Corn syrup or corn syrup solids
- Dehydrated cane juice
- Dextrin
- Dextrose
- Fructose
- Fruit juice concentrate
- Glucose
- High-fructose corn syrup
- Lactose
- Maltodextrin
- Malt syrup
- Maltose
- Rice Syrup
- Saccharose
- Sucrose
- Treacle
- Kylose

All sugar is not created equal. Raw sugar, honey, pure maple syrup are much better choices than processed sugar, but if you are trying to lose weight, any sugar will slow down the process. The body doesn't know the difference between bad sugar and better sugar – it will turn any sugar into fat.

Be aware that most processed foods that are labeled "low fat" have added sugar to adjust the taste.

Eating Tips to Make Weight Loss Easier

Eat Slowly
Savor the experience. Don't eat and run. It takes 20 minutes for your stomach to tell your brain that you are full. This will help you avoid overeating.

Drink Plenty of Water (six to eight glasses a day)
When you drink water, the body works to raise the temperature of the water and burns calories, which makes you feel full. Have plenty of bottles in the frig at home and at least a couple on your desk at work.

Have Healthy Foods Available that You Can Chew
Try apples, celery, carrots, nuts, and whole-grain hearty bread. When chewing is required, it slows down the eating process and you eat less. Watch your portions with the nuts and whole-grain bread, they are high in calories

Eat Whole Fresh Fruit Instead of Juice
Do this whenever possible. The whole fruit is more satisfying, provides much-needed fiber, and is overall more enjoyable. Never drink canned or bottled juice. There is nothing fresh about it. It is basically flavored sugar water.

If You Must Have Something Sweet . . .
Remember that your sweet craving can be satisfied without all the sugar or carbs. Experiment to find what works for you. One-fourth cup sliced berries with a dollop of Greek non-fat yogurt and a little honey drizzled on the top works great, so does a few almonds (they are quite sweet). Try an apple or banana – both sweet fruits.

Don't Starve Yourself!
If you do, your body goes into protection mode. It begins holding onto food by storing it as fat rather than burning it. This robs the muscles of the nutrients needed to stay strong.

This is the reason you should eat breakfast – to get your metabolism working and your body functioning effectively for the entire day. And, don't make a habit of skipping lunch or dinner either. An occasional missed meal is not a serious matter, but deliberately missing meals to cut calories is not a good practice.

If you don't have time to eat a full meal, at least have a healthy snack – preferably some kind of protein and a fruit or vegetable. For example: a few slices of cheese and an apple; a banana spread lightly with peanut butter; non-fat Greek yogurt with sliced strawberries – or a smoothie with a scoop of protein powder, ½ cup 2% milk and a ½ cup of frozen berries/cherries (delicious, filling, and less than 200 calories).

Have a Small, Healthy Snack Before Dinner

A bite here and there as you cook can add a lot of extra calories. Munching on celery or carrots is a great way to remove that temptation and keep you satisfied while cooking. It will also curb your hunger so you will not be tempted to overeat.

Eat Junk Food ONLY When You Prepare It Yourself!

If you must peel, chop, and deep fry potatoes every time you want French fries then you probably won't eat them very often.

The same goes for eating sweets such as chocolate cake, chocolate chip cookies, and apple pie. If you only have one piece each time you are willing to make them yourself from scratch (which ensures the use of healthy ingredients), you will automatically cut down on the frequency that you will eat them.

Make Your Changes Quietly

The decision to make a significant life change is a very personal decision. This is especially true when tackling something as challenging as changing your way of eating – especially when it includes the goal to lose weight.

Diet gurus generally advise people to set a goal and announce it to the world. They claim that it makes you accountable for your behavior. In theory, it sounds good; but, it is not.

There are several reasons why it is better to keep a lifestyle decision that involves food and weight loss to yourself.

When you choose to quietly make changes in your eating habits, you don't have to deal with pressure from friends and family. Announcing your goals to the world opens the door to everyone and their grandmother to comment about what you are eating (or not eating), and everything *they* believe you are doing wrong.

There are even "studies" often referenced by "the experts" that support the idea that the act of announcing your goals satisfies you so much emotionally that it makes you work harder on the actual nutritional aspects and exercise portion of your plan.

The studies would lead you to believe that announcing your goals is all you need to do to accomplish them. Sadly, they don't discuss the guilt and shame you feel when, after announcing them to your friends, family, co-workers, and Facebook Friends, you have to publicly admit your failure when you don't achieve your proclaimed goal of 50 pounds weight loss in 5 weeks (which, by the way, is almost impossible to do without damaging your health!)

There is no doubt that support can be a good thing, which would be the main reason for announcing your goals to the world. You hope people will cheer you on and help you get past obstacles you encounter as you change your eating habits.

Part of you may even appreciate (to a certain point) when a well-meaning loved one gives you "that look" when you load up on some fattening dessert at your mom's house.

For those of you who love and use social media regularly, PLEASE avoid the temptation to maintain a running dialog on social media about what you are, or are not, eating.

Don't get caught in the craze to use apps to tweet your progress. There are apps that will auto-Tweet your weight each week. There is another app that tells everyone on social media when you skipped a workout at the gym.

If you fall into that trap, you may as well walk around with a sign around your neck that tells everyone you meet that you need their approval to be happy.

Setting yourself up for unnecessary pressure from others *is not helpful*.

It is easy to forget that this journey toward better health is not about your friends and family – *it is about you.*

You are the only one who needs to know what you are doing. *It is your personal, private journey.*

There are a few times when it is appropriate to let others know what you are doing –and, those times occur when another person's behavior is being problematic for you.

For example, if your grandmother serves you pie every time you visit (and you visit often). You don't want to eat it, but you also don't want to hurt her feelings. You need to lovingly explain to her the journey you are on and ask her not to serve you a sweet dessert. Tell her fresh fruit, a cup of coffee, or your favorite tea would be great choices instead.

If your co-workers are continually asking you to join them for drinks and appetizers or pushing you into attending an endless stream of office celebrations with empty-calorie food and drinks, you can politely decline the invitations altogether, or choose to attend to be social and simply say "No thanks," when the drinks and food are offered.

What you ***do not need to do*** is make a loud declaration about your plan to eat healthier and/or how much weight you plan to lose, etc.

REMEMBER – this is your personal journey and your progress is no one's business except your own.

Eliminate Negative Dialogue

The way you talk to yourself and think about your daily actions can have a significant impact on your progress. You must get negative thoughts or comments such as "I cheated" or "I fell off the wagon" under control.

Negative dialogue (even with yourself) prevents you from *feeling* positive about what you are doing.

Will you occasionally make choices that are not particularly good for you? SURE!

Is that a reason to beat yourself up through negative thoughts and comments? NO! It does nothing but discourages you.

As you look at the road ahead – from this day to the rest of your life, keep in mind that every day does not have to be regimented and restricted. Eating healthy does not mean that you can never have a piece of candy again – or you can never eat dessert with your family.

You can learn to make choices that will allow you to enjoy eating, stop feeling deprived and help you live a healthy life. It is about balance and choosing foods rich in nutrients.

Once you internalize the concepts we have introduced in this book and learn to use the tools we have given you, you will be free to occasionally enjoy foods that are not part of your regular eating habits. You will be able to eat them with pleasure, with no guilt, and no raking yourself over the coals for the indulgence.

As I have explained, my journey began in January. Part of that journey included the elimination of sugar from my diet. I hadn't missed it until later in the year when the holiday season drew close.

Each day my craving for pumpkin pie grew stronger. Finally, I stopped by my favorite pie shop and bought a piece. I took it home, smothered in in whipped cream, and enjoyed every bite. It was delicious.

It satisfied my craving and I did not fall into the trap of thinking my out-of-the-ordinary choice meant that I would start eating sugar every day. Those occasional cravings can be satisfied without danger if you are very clear that it is a "one-off" choice.

In other words, a single choice to eat something that is not part of your new lifestyle does not mean you are doomed to indulge yourself every day with sweets and treats.

Leave Guilt Behind

When you are willing to stop feeling guilty about choices you make, you will see how easy it is to indulge from time to time without turning it into an official (and unhealthy) binge.

As you move forward with a clear plan to improve your way of eating in order to live a healthier life, you understand that ***reaching your goal will take as long as it takes.*** That means there are no deadlines to meet, and no one is looking over your shoulder to criticize or give advice. No reason to feel guilty about anything.

The bottom line is that when you are committed and expect success you will do your best every day to follow your plan because the future holds the promise of a healthier body and your ability to love the way you look.

You take everything in stride and at your own pace. With weight loss you know plateaus are inevitable and they sometimes last much longer than you would like; but, they don't have to derail you. You simply continue with your eating plan, expect success and feel confident that you will get past the plateau and move forward.

This is all possible with no feelings of guilt because you are answering to no one except yourself. There is no pressure and no guilt.

Chapter Eight
Move Your Body

Exercise is an important component in building a healthier body. A healthy diet by itself is not enough. If you want to live a long, healthy life, you must not only eat well, you must move your body regularly to maximize the benefits of your eating plan.

How Active Are You?

Most people think they are more active than they are, which means the majority can benefit from getting more activity each day. This is especially true if you are trying to lose weight.

You will need to know your activity level to effectively determine your required daily calorie intake to stay healthy (and to lose weight).

Using an app to track your exercise can help you identify your current activity level. If you think you fall into one of the lower levels of activity, a simple steps app would probably be adequate. If you are in one of the higher activity levels, a more advanced type of app could be a better choice.

To begin, read through the descriptions below and choose the one you think best fits your current level.

Low Movement - Sedentary

A sedentary or inactive lifestyle means that you have no formal exercise routine and are not physically active during the day. Sedentary people are known to have what is called the "sitting disease." That is all they do – sit. They may get up to go to the restroom, their bed, or the kitchen – but other than that, they are essentially "couch potatoes."

A sedentary lifestyle contributes to weight gain and eventually, obesity. It decreases the sense of overall well-being and can increase the risk of developing certain health problems and diseases, such heart issues and Type 2 diabetes.

For some people, this is not a choice. You may be recovering from a serious illness or injury that restricts your movement. In these situations, it is wise to follow doctor's orders, rest, and heal. When the time is right, gradually increase your level of activity as health permits.

If you fall into this category and ***are not*** constrained for health reasons, ***it is time*** to increase your activity level and improve your health.

Being *home* all day doesn't necessarily mean you are sedentary – even if you happen to sit quite a bit. If you are active around the house during the day – cooking, cleaning, gardening, working in the garage, etc., you may belong in the next level of movement.

If you are not sure whether you are "Sedentary" or the next level up - "Light Movement," track your movement for two or three weeks; but, make sure they are typical and not weeks of unusual activities that require more movement than normal.

Also, keep a record of the time you spend sitting – and what you are doing. Are you sitting very still, staring out the window? Reading a good book? Playing video games? Watching a good TV show or movie?

The goal is to eventually incorporate more physical movement into some of your favorite activities that may tend to be sedentary. For example, there are video game consoles like Kinect that require movement so you are not being sedentary at all.

Light Movement

Light movement includes more movement than a sedentary person; but, it is a long way from hardcore exercise. The light mover doesn't always consciously include exercise in their daily routine. Often it is the result of their ordinary responsibilities and schedule.

People who fall under this category could be college students who walk from class to class and across campus, people who work in an office and are constantly getting up and down out of their chairs, or workers who have jobs where they are continually moving such as doctors, nurses, and blue-collar laborers (although some fall into the next category).

Light physical activity can also include activities done as part of everyday life, such as walking your dog twice a day; sweeping, mopping, and vacuuming; gardening; or playing catch with your kids.

These types of activities typically burn about 150 calories a day for the average person. But the number of calories can vary greatly depending on your body size and the specific type and duration of the activity.

When you start tracking your movement, you may be surprised how much you move daily. If you are clocking 120-180 minutes of light exercise each week, you fall into the "Light Movement" category even if you are not working up a complete sweat when you exercise.

The following are examples of light physical activity
- Walking slowly (15-20 Minutes/3Xs week)
- Raking leaves
- Casually shooting baskets
- Sitting using the computer (stand-up breaks are important)
- Standing light work (cooking, washing dishes, sweeping, mopping)
- Playing most musical instruments

Although these are not extended exercise routines, exercise of any kind has benefits – better cholesterol levels, reduced body fat, improved blood pressure, and improved metabolic health.

Those who are lightly active rather than sedentary also experience improved quality of life and typically have a lower risk of developing chronic disease.

Moderate Movement

This would include some type of moderate cardio/respiratory exercise for 20 to 60 minutes, three to five days a week. It could be Jazzercize, aerobics, running/jogging or jumping rope. (There are many others). Your moderate physical activity may also include strength training and stretching exercises and family fun time.

Examples of exercise - three to five times a week.
- Brisk walking (30 minutes, 4 mph)
- Heavy cleaning (washing windows, vacuuming, mopping)
- Mowing lawn (power mower)
- Bicycling light effort (10-12 mph)
- Bad Minton recreational
- Tennis doubles
- Running for 30 minutes
- Jogging for 30 minutes
- Elliptical workout for 20 minutes

Moderate physical routines provide all the benefits of light physical routines plus they gain the benefits of increased heart health, increased muscular strength and greater endurance and flexibility – plus, an improvement in overall health, quality of life, and less risk of chronic disease risk.

Vigorous Movement

Exercise enthusiasts are those who are extremely active. These people not only get movement throughout their day due to basic decisions like walking to deliver a message instead of emailing; they also work in a regular solid exercise routine that gets their hearts beating before each day is done.

This level includes regular vigorous exercise for 20 to 60 minutes almost every day – some take one day off each week. Their routines are usually a combination of cardio, strength training, and aerobics.

Example: They vigorously exercise daily, participating in of any of the following, plus others that they enjoy.
- Hiking
- Shoveling snow
- Lifting and carrying heavy boxes all day
- Swimming laps
- High-intensity aerobics
- Weight training
- Running and jogging
- Rock climbing
- Singles tennis
- Swing dancing

Vigorous exercise routines provide all the benefits of light and moderate activities; plus, there is an even greater reduction in chronic disease risk.

These are people who fall into the athletic category. If you regularly play a sport or participate in athletic events like continual training for marathons, you are vigorously active.

Some careers require extreme physical activity – such as the military, some agriculture laborers, USPS/FedEx delivery men/women, and other industrial workers.

If you are physically active for six to 10 hours or more a week, you would be considered extremely active.

It is important to be aware that a vigorous exercise routine carries a greater risk of injury and possible burnout from overtraining. If this is your choice, we recommend that you check with your doctor before starting such an intensive program.

Summary

All movement is good for you. Take the time to tally up the hours to determine your current activity level – and where you want to be in the future. Enter your findings in the ***Introspective Evaluation.***

Then, you can develop an eating plan that helps you fuel your body properly. The last thing you want is to cut calories to such a deficit that you weaken your energy supply and become ***less active*** and less able to reach your healthy weight goal.

Chapter Nine

Natural Ways to Burn More Calories

There are many ways you can go from sedentary to light movement, to moderate or even to a vigorous exercise enthusiast. You can join classes for fitness, invest in exercise equipment, or commit to a regimented program that will get you moving more.

I applaud you if you choose any of those, but the best way to approach the change is to identify where you are currently and move up one level at a time in order to allow your body to adjust to the changes and ensure long-term success.

Don't push your body beyond healthy limits. Unless your level of exercise is already moderate to vigorous, a smart choice would be to simply increase your average, everyday activities.

You do not have to be an exercise fanatic to get results. Gradually increasing daily physical activities can quickly add up and result in better health.

Use an Activity Tracker

If you don't have time to set up a daily exercise routine, you can still burn calories by walking and track your efforts by using a step-tracker. The choices today are endless. You can choose from a simple ***pedometer*** to a ***FitBit*** to a complex ***Apple Watch***. The choices range in price from $20 to several hundred dollars.

The least expensive choice is a simple pedometer/activity tracker. The ***Omron HJ-203 Pedometer with Activity Tracker*** sells for less than $20 and tracks steps, distance, calories and fat grams. It includes a clock, is smaller than a credit card, and comes with a strap or clip for easy attachment to your clothes.

Other choices range from simple step counters to more complicated trackers that record health information and track exercise routines separately.

Or - if you have a Smart Phone, there are free apps you can install to track almost anything you choose. I use the **Pedometer ++** app to track my steps *(walking is my preferred form of exercise.)*

Studies show that using a tracker helps people on their weight-loss journey because you can see the results of your hard work and easily check your daily progress. Walking 10,000 steps just going about your daily routine is equivalent to walking five miles.

I started with the pedometer and graduated to the iPhone Watch that now does the job for me. I hate keeping records, so a tracker is "pure gold" in my eyes.

Once you get started you may be inspired to look for ways to add to your step count, such as parking further away from the door of the store when you go shopping; and climbing stairs at work rather than take the elevator.

Set a daily goal. If you are not used to doing anything physical, start slowly and increase your progress a little each day you meet or exceed the goal. After a week or so at that level, challenge yourself with a new goal.

When you eat a healthy diet and use a tracker regularly, you will enjoy seeing those pounds fall off and feel better, as well.

Short Bursts of Exercise at Work

Even if you sit at a desk all day, you can still get in some quick and effective moves that will help you stay fit.

Brisk Walks - Go for lunch walks or break walks. If you don't have the time to get outside at your office, walk the halls of your office area. Walk to deliver messages personally instead of using email.

Use the Stairs – Instead of using the elevator, take the stairs. For every flight you climb, the calories are burning, your heart is pumping and the steps are adding up.

Get Rid of Your Desk Chair and sit on a large exercise ball. Using an exercise ball strengthens your abdominal muscles and your calf muscles at the same time.

Seated Leg Lifts - Simply lift your left leg and hold it out straight with your foot flexed back toward your body. Count to ten and lower the leg slowly. Switch to the right leg and do the same. Alternate each leg for ten repetitions each to tighten those muscles.

Standing Leg Lifts – These can be done almost anywhere; for example: standing at the water machine, in the elevator, while talking on the phone, or waiting for someone in your office. Stand on one leg and bend the other one at the knee so that you are raising the heel of your foot toward your rear end. Hold until the count of ten then slowly put your foot down; repeat with the other leg.

Use Hand Weights – Small dumbbells that come in all sizes are a great choice for people who are on the phone a lot.

Be sure to choose a good weight for you. The <u>Mayo Clinic</u> says the correct weight for you should be the one that is heavy enough to tire your muscles after about 12 to 15 repetitions. You should be just barely able to finish the last repetition.

You should practice with these at home. Learn how to use them properly and get comfortable using them – then take them to the office. Don't hurt yourself.

Toe Raises – These can be done sitting at your desk. With the heel of your foot on the ground, lift the toes of your foot upward and hold for the count of ten. Lower your foot and switch to the other foot. Repeat at least 10 times each.

Squeeze Your Glutes - Burn calories and get your rear in shape at the same time by squeezing your glutes. You can do this at your desk, while you are waiting to go into a meeting, or even get in a few quick squeezes while in the restroom.

Pushups and Situps – These are good choices if you have an area where you can be alone for a few minutes. Do some pushups on the floor or against the wall. Not a big fan of pushups? Try situps instead – or do both.

Jumping Jacks, *Running in Place*, and *Walking Lunges* are all quick and easy exercises that can be done at the office in a somewhat private area or outdoors during your break or lunch – a couple of minutes at a time several times throughout the day can easily add up to a good workout.

These are only a few of the possibilities. There are many more options that you will discover as you get going.

House Cleaning Is a Physical Activity

Sometimes, there is simply no time to get to the gym or to go for a walk because life is too busy - or maybe you would rather do anything other than commit to a daily exercise routine. However, you do not want to lose the momentum you have going and believe there must be other ways to help you burn calories. Guess what . . . there are!

Whenever your body is in motion, it is burning calories. If you don't have time to exercise or you hate to exercise, then start cleaning!

Check out all the calories you can burn in one hour by just doing what must be done around the home: Sweeping floors (156 calories), mopping (170 calories), vacuuming (170 calories), washing dishes (88 calories), dusting (85 calories), sweeping the garage and sidewalks (204 calories), etc.

If you worked for a half hour making the bed, dusting the room, and vacuuming, you would burn a total of 112 calories. If it took you an hour, you would double that number. Before you clean your bedroom, if you decide to do some laundry first, you will burn 17 calories for every 15 minutes you spend doing laundry.

Spring cleaning your house burns even more calories. In fact, it can give you the same vigorous workout you would get if you were going hard at it on a treadmill. Doing simple chores burns calories, too. Clearing the table and washing the dishes, uses 50 calories.

Chores, where you work up a sweat, can really take off the calories. If you need to clean your bathroom, you will burn 100 calories every half hour you devote to it. If you live in a home that has more than one bathroom, you get to multiply that loss by the number of bathrooms you have for every half hour that you clean.

The best part about knocking off calories through cleaning your house (besides having a clean house at the end of all the chores) is that it does not have to be done all at once the way you would complete a workout at the gym.

Instead of spending hours cleaning, you can clean in short bursts for 10-15 minutes at a time throughout the day and still get the same benefit you would if you had worked straight through.

Be sure to add a little fun in the mix. Take your dog for a walk around your neighborhood. Depending on your weight, you can easily burn 150 calories or more for every half hour you spend walking your pet.

Burn off 136 calories dancing with a broom. Remember the wise word of Snow White, "Whistle while you work."

Yard Work Will Burn More Calories

The things you do to make the outside of your house look nice can be a good way for you to exercise as well. Washing the outside windows of your home knocks off 102 calories in a thirty-minute time span and will make your house sparkle!

Mowing the lawn is an outside activity that will burn calories fast. If you weigh 200 pounds, or more, you can burn over 276 calories for each half an hour it takes you to mow. So, if you mow for an hour, you will burn over 550 calories.

Washing your car can burn up to 204 or more calories every hour. If you like flower gardening, you can have a yard filled with pretty flowers and take off 272 calories for every hour you spend giving your home some curb appeal.

Fun Activities Burn Calories

Burning calories doesn't all have to be chore related. Fun physical activities that help you relax can also burn calories. Dancing is one that I personally love. You can dance at home, with friends, or in an organized group class. It can be ballroom, swing, or aerobic – dancing is dancing.

Wherever you choose to dance, you will spin and burn those calories away. Dancing can burn 240 or more calories per half hour depending on the type of dancing that is involved. More complex moves and faster rhythms produce greater results. Enjoy and dance at your own pace – it all helps.

Many people enjoy roller skating or ice skating, which can easily burn 350 or more calories for every half an hour that you spend doing it.

A kickboxing class could burn 960 calories in one hour. Not only are you getting fit, but you could also be learning some helpful self-defense moves at the same time.

Racquet games such as tennis, badminton or squash are faster-paced and burn more calories. Squash burns the most, coming in at 533 calories for every half hour spent.

Tennis burns almost 400 and badminton 285. Bowling takes off 308 calories for every hour. You do not move as fast with golf, but you can walk up to five miles playing one round of 18 holes! (No golf carts allowed.)

There are some days when you don't feel like doing anything outside or inside the house, even if it is fun. On days like that, if you spend half an hour playing with your children or with your pets, you can still burn calories.

So, don't forget to enjoy yourself and remember the exercise that you get is a fringe benefit.

For more information on calories burned for a specific activity, go to **_CalorieLab.com_**.

Chapter Ten

Putting It All Together

Your New Healthy Lifestyle

If you have read each of the preceding chapters and completed the exercises, a clear picture should be developing of your new way of eating.

1. You have identified the foods you enjoy and want to keep eating.
2. You have identified foods that you want to eliminate or limit.
3. You understand the importance of nutrients, calories, and portion control.
4. You know what your daily calorie intake should be to maintain weight, to lose weight, and to lose weight fast.
5. You are fully aware of dietary requirements in connection with your health issues.
6. You know healthy foods are the best path to weight loss.
7. You have identified your current activity level and how to sustain or raise it.

It's time to implement your new lifestyle

Eat Healthy, Natural Foods

Healthy eating means eating nutritionally-rich food that will help you feel good, have lots of energy, help you reach and sustain a healthy weight for your body structure, reduce your chance of poor health and disease, and enjoy a more positive outlook (stable moods).

The foundation of your plan should be to always buy fresh organic (if possible), close-to-nature foods; eliminate processed, additive-filled foods and learn to prepare your meals in the healthiest way possible.

Growing public demand has made healthy, additive-free food and affordable organic produce readily available in most grocery stores, making it easier to eat well than it has ever been.

Now, it is up to the individual. ***You can choose to eat well, or not.***

In the beginning, when you are learning how to choose the best foods for building and maintaining a healthy body, it may seem like a lot to take in: but, it gets easier with time.

If you can practice patience, look forward to each new day as an adventure, and enjoy the delicious, healthy food you are putting into your body, you will be surprised how everything changes – your ease with the process, the way you are feeling, and your weight.

You will wake up one day and realize that you are no longer "trying" to eat well, it has become your "way of life."

Experiment and find out which foods and eating patterns work best for you. Start slowly and gradually change your old unhealthy habits. Be committed to living a healthier life.

Guidelines for Establishing a Healthy Way of Eating

- Begin with small steps ***(don't try to change everything at once).***
- Know your personal required calorie count and stay within the recommended count in order to meet your goals.
- Practice portion control - Moderation is key ***(Don't overeat and don't starve yourself).***
- Focus on eating nutrient-rich foods throughout the day.
  - Eat lots of vegetables and a couple of servings of fruit each day.
    - Frozen vegetables and fruits are acceptable substitutes for fresh - make sure you buy flash-frozen fresh veggies or fruits with no additives. *(Flash-frozen*

immediately after being harvested suspends "aging" and nutrient loss.)

- Eat whole, unrefined grains.
- Eat plenty of fiber.
- Eat only healthy fats (no more than 10% of daily calorie intake).
- Eat a little protein at each meal—including breakfast—stay with the leanest and healthiest forms. *(Remember it doesn't have to be meat.)*

- ***Eliminate all processed foods from your diet*** – including all white flour and white sugar products.
- ***Eliminate all foods with additives, preservatives, and added sugars.***
- If you must have a sweetener with your smoothies or morning coffee, use Stevia products, local organic honey, or pure maple syrup.
- Drink lots of water. ***(Staying hydrated is critical for cleansing the body.)***
- Listen to your body. ***(Eat when hungry/Stop when full.)***

Don't have a long list of "off limit" foods. That just makes you want them more. If you crave sweet, salty, or unhealthy foods, start moving away from them slowly by reducing the portion size and eating them less frequently.

As your diet begins to shift and you gradually eat less and less of the unhealthy foods, your cravings will diminish. You will be able to eat them from time to time and think of them as nothing more than an occasional indulgence.

Remember that even though you may be taking baby steps in changing your eating habits, every step counts. Every change (no matter how small) makes a difference and makes you healthier.

Small Changes Make Eating Healthy Easier

Keep Healthy Food Readily Available
When you get hungry, it is easy to eat the first thing you see on the counter or in the cupboard. Keep healthy food accessible and visible in your home and workplace.

Put some fruits in a basket on the kitchen counter, store healthy snacks at eye level in your pantry, and stock up your fridge with small batches of cooked whole grains, fresh fruits, and ready-to-eat vegetables. At work, keep small plastic bags of almonds, pistachios and dried berries on your desk or in your top drawer.

Plan Your Meals

Learning to eat healthy takes practice. You will be more successful, at first, if you plan your food for each day. This allows you to go about your day without thinking about what or when you are going to eat and how hungry you are. (This is especially important if you are trying to lose weight).

When you plan and eat healthy meals with the appropriate calorie count, the weight loss will happen naturally.

Plan for Breakfast
Breakfast does what it says – it breaks your fast. It gets your metabolism running and helps the body burn fat all day long. When you don't plan for breakfast, the morning rush creates stress on your body and leads to poor food choices.

A tip for planning breakfast is to take everything out the night before, like utensils, cereal, and anything else that can be left out on the counter; and, consolidate cold ingredients in one place in the fridge. This will help you function more efficiently in the morning.

For breakfast protein, you may want to consider some of the following: natural peanut or almond butter on a slice of whole wheat toast, Greek yogurt with berries and a teaspoon of honey, or a couple of hard-boiled eggs with your morning coffee. Eggs can be boiled the night before, shelled and placed in a Ziplock® bag in the fridge.

Morning coffee is perfectly acceptable, I even drink mine with two tablespoons of half-and-half (40 calories) and a couple of drops of Stevia for sweetener. Just be sure to include the cream in your calorie count.

Prepare Your Snacks

When you prepare your snacks the night before, it is much easier to stay on track. When you munch on a small handful of nuts, an apple/orange/banana, cherry tomatoes with hummus, a cheese stick, a cup of plain popcorn, or other healthy options from home, you will be able to satisfy hunger between meals and avoid the break room goodies and the vending machines.

Keep your snacks under 100 calories each and plan for no more than two each day for a total of 200 calories (that includes an evening snack if you plan on having one.) Also – only eat snacks if you are hungry. Don't eat a snack just because you have always eaten one at a certain time of the day.

Plan for Lunch and Dinner

When you don't have a plan for regular meals, you may end up foraging in the fridge and eating a big bowl of leftover mashed potatoes for dinner. Or worse yet, in desperation ordering pizza or driving through McDonald's. Doing that once in a great while is not a problem, but if it happens frequently, your plan for eating healthy will quickly become a good idea that never comes to fruition.

When you plan, you have a much better chance of staying on track and reaching your goals – including weight loss.

Remember – *always thoughtfully CHOOSE the foods you eat* – rather than grabbing what is available or the most convenient. If you fall into old, unhealthy eating habits regularly just because you don't plan well, you will be sabotaging your new way of life.

Fall in Love with Leftovers

If you work you probably don't have time to cook fresh meals every day of the week. I live alone so I don't enjoy cooking for one. Plus, I work full-time, go to the gym regularly, work on my writing, and keep up with the general activities of daily life. I don't have a lot of time, nor do I want to be cooking full meals every day.

Since I plan my meals – part of the planning is to make enough of some dishes to last for more than just one sitting. I usually have leftovers of at least one dish each week that will last two or three days. That is a reward for me because it means an extra easy meal (or two).

I don't mind eating the same thing more than once. Sometimes, I simply warm it up or even eat it cold in a salad. Other times, I will toss it in a frying pan with a little olive oil, a few spices and some veggies (which may be fresh or leftover, as well) and it is a new, tasty dish.

Do Not Skip Meals

Some of the current experts disagree. Some say that if you are not hungry – do not eat! This can be dangerous on so many levels. It is too easy to binge eat after skipping a meal or gravitate toward sugary, fatty, convenience foods. Also, when you do not feed your body regularly, it can go into starvation mode and store calories as fat rather than burn them, which can stall your weight loss.

A better piece of advice would be to follow your body's hunger cues – *eat when you are hungry and stop when you are full!* (You don't have to clean your plate).

Intermittent Fasting

Intermittent fasting is a new trend. There are mixed opinions about whether it is helpful or harmful. Devout members of the Mormon Church have been practicing a one-day monthly fast for almost two centuries with no bad side-effects.

Giving your body a monthly rest may be a good idea. Beyond that, I'm not so sure regular fasting (which can be taken to an extreme) is something I would choose to practice.

When it comes to skipping breakfast – it's not a great idea. If you are not particularly hungry in the morning, at least eat something to get your body started for the day ahead.

Have a piece of whole-grain toast with peanut butter, ½ cup cottage cheese with ½ sliced banana, an apple, or grapes. Have a piece of fresh fruit, a glass of freshly-squeezed orange juice, or a cup of non-fat Greek yogurt with a little honey for sweetener or topped with a tablespoon of whole-grain granola.

Big healthy breakfasts are wonderful if you enjoy them and can afford the large calorie count, but they are not necessary.

Don't forget to drink a big glass of water every morning to rehydrate your body.

Focus on What You Can Eat
Don't focus on what you must give up. For example, think about the wonderful rainbow of fruits and vegetables you can add into your diet each day for color, flavor, texture, and nutrients.

Be adventurous and try at least one new fruit or vegetable each week that you have never tried before.

Enough Said - It's Time to Begin

This book has given you a great deal of information and you may be a little overwhelmed. However, I want to assure you that establishing a healthy diet and reaping the benefits from the added nutrition you can receive is not difficult. You simply make it happen.

As I have mentioned before, grocery stores are beginning to stock a wide selection of fresh, organic foods, cage-free eggs, grain-fed beef and even some packaged goods that are not filled with additives (although, I still recommend that you stay away from packaged goods as much as possible.)

Eating well does not require buying "superfoods" and expensive products to get the necessary nutrients.

When I talk to people about upgrading their diets to healthier foods, they often complain that they will be stuck with the same few foods repeatedly, which would be horrible. But, that is a needless fear.

If you were to conduct a study, you would find that most families eat the same 12 to 14 meals every month, year-after-year. They are in a recycle mode that rarely includes anything new.

If that is true of your family – don't worry about it; but, my guess is that once you discover the wide-variety of nutritious fresh foods available, you will be introducing more variety – not less – into your diet.

Eating well can be a fun adventure filled with colorful, delicious food that is exciting and enjoyable – far from boring.

How to Proceed

Use all the knowledge and information you have gathered from the book and get started on your new way of eating. You have all the information you need to be successful.

- You understand nutrients.
- You have a list of nutrient-filled foods that you like.
- You have a list of foods that you are going to eliminate or limit.
- Your long-term goal has been clearly defined and written down.
- You have accepted that *it will take as much time as it takes to reach the goal.*
- You have recorded your beginning weight.
- You know what your daily calorie intake is going to be.
- You have smaller plates and understand portion control – with a good idea of what a healthy portion is.
- You have an app on your phone (or computer) so you can track your calorie intake each time you eat.
- You have set your exercise goal and you have an app to track it, as well.
- You know how many hours of sleep you need each night.

On Your Mark! Get Set! GO!

Step #1 - Clean out your refrigerator and pantry

Toss out all processed foods (or give it away) – this includes everything made with white flour and sugar. If that is too painful, set a start date for your new way of eating and get rid of a little bit at a time . . . and DON'T buy any more.

Stock only healthy, nutritious food. Do not keep unhealthy foods around to tempt you or your children.

If you are committed to eating well, you must take this step.

Step #2 - Create a menu for Week One – If you are inspired you can also plan for Week Two

Then, make your shopping list for the first week.

After you have ***finished a good lunch***, go shopping for Week One ***(never shop when you are hungry).***

You will find that grocery shopping is easier when you are not buying processed foods because there are fewer sections to visit and no labels to read. In fact, you will find that most of the foods you want are placed around the perimeter of the store.

When you are ready to shop for Week Two, either create your menu or make necessary changes to the menu you created with Week One. Then, complete your shopping list and buy your groceries for Week Two.

You may have some food leftover from Week One that can be incorporated into your Week Two menu so it can be crossed off the shopping list; or, you may have missed something important the first week that you need to pick up.

When it comes to planning and shopping, you will find your own rhythm. It is much easier for me to plan for a few days or one week at a time. After a few weeks, you will find what works best for you.

Step #3 – Remember the 80/20 Rule

Changing your eating habits can be challenging. I recommend that you apply the 80/20 rule. Your effort to eat well should be right on target at least 80% of the time – and you may slip 20% of the time.

Don't beat yourself up when you slip. But, acknowledge your actions and think about how you can avoid the slip in the future. Even doing everything perfectly 80% of the time will bring great results.

Slowly, but surely, you want to increase your percentage up to 100%; but in the beginning, if you are consistently at 80%, you are doing well.

You may even be surprised at the changes in how you feel (mentally and physically) and in your increased energy levels as you embrace the adventure of eating well-balanced, nutritious meals.

Step #4 - Enjoy eating

Food sustains life and should be enjoyed and shared with love. Eat with family or friends whenever you have the chance.

Even if you are alone, set a nice place at the table, enjoy a small glass of red wine, relax, and savor the amazing flavors and textures of the food you are eating. Mealtime should be pleasant and enjoyable – something to look forward to.

Eating well is not about deprivation, it is about abundance – enjoying nature's harvest.

If you are basically healthy (with no serious health issues), your new way of eating will eliminate restrictions and constant worry over what you should, or should not, eat. Tasty, delicious meals, good health, and a sense of well-being will be the norm.

Step #5 – Exercise regularly

Remember it doesn't have to be a lot; but, it should be consistent.

Determine how physically active you are currently and increase your exercise gradually to a level that your body can sustain.

Step #6 - Get enough sleep

The average person needs between seven and nine hours each night. If for some reason that is not possible because of your responsibilities, incorporate "power naps" into your daily routine to avoid sleep deprivation.

It Is Time to Get Started!

Expect Success

Implement your new plan with ***the expectation of success.***

There may be that pesky niggle at the back of your mind saying, "You have failed before, you will probably fail again."

That does not have to be true. However, if you buy into it and believe you will fail, chances are you will! A failure mindset dramatically increases your chances for failure. It will be impossible to develop a sustainable healthy lifestyle because there is no true commitment in place.

Expecting success involves seeing a clear picture of yourself healthier, more energetic, and trimmer than ever before based on what you plan to do – and continue to do, day-after-day.

An expectation of success demands dedicated focus and doing what you must to succeed – which is where your personal evaluation comes in to play. The summary of your findings will clarify what you need to do – it should be your roadmap.

If you are ***100% convinced right now*** that if you stay with your new way of healthy eating, push yourself to establish a regular exercise routine, and get enough sleep, you will lose every pound of weight that you want to lose and become a healthier, trimmer YOU because of your efforts.

It is time to ***expect success***.

Chapter Eleven

What About Supplements?

Hopefully, you have made the decision to establish a new healthier lifestyle, rather than simply "go on a diet" to lose weight. It will be an exciting journey; but, before you begin, there is one more thing we need to discuss.

You have done your homework and chosen a diet plan that fits your needs and will put you soundly on the road to good health. You have also developed a sustainable activity schedule that works for you. The last thing to consider is . . . do you need to take any supplements?

The supplement industry rakes in billions of dollars every year. New health companies spring up daily and promote their superfoods, vitamins, and supplements through every advertising medium. Their products are sold in multiple outlets, from the Internet to the local grocery stores.

This vast availability of supplements raises the question: Should you take the easy path and load your body with supplements, superfoods, powdered "smoothie" concoctions or is it possible (and better) to get enough of the critical nutrients from regular food?

There is an abundance of advice on supplements – much of it conflicting, so how can you make a good decision?

The best advice is to ask your doctor. What does s/he recommend based on the current state of your health, and your family history so that you can prevent future problems.

Most people understand that getting enough vitamins and minerals in their diets is fundamental to good health; but despite that knowledge, many people are deficient. What is the best way to ensure that your body is getting adequate amounts?

Nutritionists always recommend that you eat a healthy diet in order to get the nutrients you need from real food, not from supplements. No one would recommend that you live on energy drinks, convenience foods and a handful of pills each day. That would be absurd . . . and yet, there are people who try to do just that.

A Healthy Diet Is the Best Choice

It is possible to get all the vitamins and minerals the body needs from food if you are smart about your choices.

The healthiest diet you can choose is made up of mostly plants and organic grass-fed, free-range animal products that are void of hormones and additives. With this kind of diet, you will consume enough nutrients in your food that supplements will be unnecessary.

If you want to be sure if you should take any supplements, ask your doctor to test your blood serum levels for vitamin and mineral deficiencies. In fact, you should have this done as part of your annual physical.

Nutrition from the food you eat is, by far, the best way to improve your health – both short-term and long-term. Pills and potions (supplements) can only do so much. Even with them, if you continue to eat empty-calorie foods that are filled with additives and devoid of nutrition, your health will suffer.

A healthy diet as described above should be enough to build and sustain a strong healthy body, but there are a few situations which may require supplements.

When Supplements Are Needed

Vitamin B12 Deficiency
There are some people who lack an enzyme that helps them metabolize Vitamin B12. The only way to know if you are one of those people is to be tested. If you are deficient, you should take a Vitamin B12 supplement. The easiest way is through injections given by your doctor.

B12 deficiency is a serious issue that can cause long-term neurological disorders. As a point of information, most vegans find they need to supplement vitamin B12.

Vitamin D Deficiency
Most people do not spend enough time out in the sun, and even those who do use heavy sunscreen due to cancer fears, plus the average person takes a daily shower. As a result, it is difficult for our bodies to make enough vitamin D, specifically D2 and D3. It is important to get your levels checked and supplement, if needed. However, sunlight and food are still the best sources of Vitamin D (AKA the "Sunshine Vitamin").

Your body is designed to get the Vitamin D it needs by producing it when your bare skin is exposed to sunlight – when the sun is high in the sky. The most effective time for this exposure is at noon when the ultraviolet B (UVB) rays can do their job.

Exposure to direct sunlight does not have to be extended. In fact, if you live in the UK, 13 minutes of sunlight exposure around noon three times each week is enough to maintain healthy levels among light-skinned adults.

Recently, an international team of researchers from the University of Exeter Medical School in England released results from a study that indicated Vitamin D deficiency substantially increases the risk of dementia and Alzheimer's disease.

Other studies have shown that the sunshine vitamin also protects against a host of other diseases, including osteoporosis, heart disease, and breast, prostate and colon cancers. In addition to disease prevention, sunlight has several hidden benefits – like protection against depression, insomnia, and an overactive immune system.

A Word of Caution

As we discussed, your diet must take into consideration your health issues and medications you may be taking. You must be careful about what you eat and the supplements you take. ***Be aware of possible interactions that may occur.***

For example: When taking cholesterol medications (statins), you should avoid eating grapefruit as part of your diet. According to the <u>U.S. Food and Drug Administration</u>, it can affect the rate at which drugs are processed by the liver, which can be dangerous. A slower breakdown of the drug could result in too much of the drug in your bloodstream at one time.

St. John's Wort is another common supplement that has potentially serious interactions with some prescription drugs. According to Web M.D., it interacts with Alprazolam, Amitriptyline, birth control pills, Digoxin, and others.

The bottom line is to eat a good healthy diet, have your blood tested annually for vitamin and mineral deficiencies and take supplements as needed (and recommended by your doctor) to keep your blood serum levels where they should be for good health.

Do NOT self-medicate!

Chapter Twelve

Milestones

If weight loss is one of your primary goals, curiosity and concern may drive you to weigh-in daily. My recommendation (if you can manage it) is to restrain yourself and weigh-in once a week. For example, every Sunday morning – and enter the result on your app. This will give you a visual of how things are going.

Daily weigh-ins are not recommended because the natural fluctuation of your weight can be discouraging if you are trying to lose pounds. Your primary focus should be on your lifestyle change, not an obsession with pounds lost (or not lost).

Regardless of how frequently you weigh-in and whatever the result, do not be discouraged – weight is very dynamic and will fluctuate. If it goes up a pound . . . remember, if you stay on track, it will go down a pound, plus more. The important daily check-in is with yourself and how you are feeling today.

Tracking for the Long-Term

When you are implementing a long-term plan for a healthier lifestyle, it is wise to use monthly, quarterly, and semi-annual, or annual check-ins to ensure you are on the right track.

Monthly Check-ins

Keep a record of your findings as you go along and summarize at the end of every month to determine how you are doing. There is a chart in the *Introspective Evaluation* to make this easier. But remember, numbers are only one measure. It is also important to evaluate how you are feeling.

When you are in tune with your body, you can usually tell how well you have done during the month by the way you feel. If you are feeling tired or run down, you may not be getting all the nutrients you need. If you are energized and feeling great physically and mentally, you are probably right on track.

However, just-in-case, check your tracker to be sure you are eating enough of the right foods – foods that are nutrient- rich and contain an adequate calorie count for you to stay healthy. If you discover an area that is lacking, ***make the necessary adjustments.***

If you can't figure out what is missing, ask your doctor to do a simple blood test to tell you what you should add to your diet. Remember that too much of some vitamins or minerals can potentially also have negative effects - just as too little can. So, it is important to pay attention to what you have been eating (or not eating).

Keep a record of your weight loss. The rate at which you are losing weight is also an indication of whether, or not, you are getting enough nutrients. If you start to lose weight too fast (more than 2 pounds a week) that is a sign that you are not replacing the fuel that your body is burning.

For a truly healthy lifestyle, healthy eating should always be accompanied by regular exercise. This is even more important if weight-loss is part of your goal.

If you are not exercising enough, you may hit a weight-loss plateau (you aren't gaining, but you are also not losing weight). When that happens, you may need to step up the exercise a bit.

A regular exercise routine helps you lose the weight, but it also helps tone areas of your body that need toning – plus it keeps your organs healthy. However, do not overdo it. You do not want to push your body to the extent that you are straining and spraining your body.

Too much exercise will cause you to lose too much weight and will send your body into starvation mode. When that happens, your metabolism slows down as part of your body's safety mechanism. You do not want that to happen because a slower metabolism makes losing weight more difficult.

Stepping onto the scale during regular weigh-ins helps track your progress. Stay within healthy parameters for weight loss. ***Doctors recommend no more than 1-2 pounds a week.*** Any faster after the initial first week is too fast.

If you are not losing enough, check your eating patterns, your daily calorie count, your portions, and increase your exercise a little.

Don't drop into an emotional pit when your weight plateaus or increases a pound or two. Weight will fluctuate! It is normal.

Notice how your clothes fit and check your body's measurements every month. Measure your chest area, your waist and hips to see if those numbers are going down. ***Clothing fit and measurements are usually better indicators of weight loss than the scale.***

Quarterly Check-ins

With any new weight loss and fitness journey, as you near the end of the first quarter, enthusiasm may begin to lag. This can be the result of several things, but it is usually because you have fallen into a rut.
-    You have been using the same exercise routine for too long.
-    You always eat the same food without any variation – there is nothing new to look forward to.

Since this is a long-term journey, it is important to switch things up a bit from time to time, so that your diet and exercise do not become boring and stagnant. Every quarter (three months) is a good time to take a serious look at your routine and consciously make changes.

If you started at the beginning of the year and have been stuck inside because of the weather, with the arrival of spring you can start enjoying the fresh air again and go for a run or walk each day.

Summer requires a different type of exercise to replace running during the hot months. It is a great time to sign up for a vigorous indoor dance class or a martial arts class to move your body.

If you are used to exercising alone and feel the need for accountability and motivation, consider getting an exercise partner or personal trainer.

You also want to check to see what it is that your body is saying to you. How do your skin and hair look? If you are eating well and getting enough exercise, your skin and hair will reflect the benefits. If your skin is dry and your hair is dull and lackluster, you will need to make adjustments.

After three months, some of your pesky problem areas should have shown signs of change (for the better). If you have not noticed any changes by the end of the first quarter, you must adjust your nutritional intake and physical activity to find what works for you.

In the first quarter, your body should have changed in some way. Your skin is looking healthier, inches have been lost, your body may be a little firmer than before, and your *BMI number should have improved – at least a little* (don't worry if it is not a big change yet). Go to **BMICalculator.cc** to calculate your Body Mass Index.

Also, look at your weight loss goals. See if you are where you wanted to be since you started your journey. If you are not where you wanted to be – remember, ***"It will take as long as it takes."***

Celebrate your efforts and what you have accomplished. Seeing progress, even in small increments, can help you stick with it for the long haul. Remember – it is okay to make changes. What worked for you in the beginning may not work for you now. It is okay to change your diet (if the

changes are healthy), your routine - *and* your goals, if necessary. The goal
is for you to get healthy – and stay healthy! And . . . it may take longer
than you want it to. So be patient.

Semi-annual or Annual Check-ups

A semi-annual or an annual check-up is very important when you are on a
weight loss, get-fit-for-life journey. Seeing positive changes on the
outside does not always indicate that internal changes are where they
need to be.

The only way that you can tell if everything is going well inside is to have
your doctor check your progress. He or she can run a blood panel to
verify that your numbers are good or improving.

If you are diabetic or pre-diabetic, of course, you want to get your
glucose level tested for current levels; and, you will also want an A1c test
to tell you if your glucose levels were within range for the previous three
months.

Everyone should have cholesterol tested as well. If you struggle with high
cholesterol, it should go down with the right diet. Once again, you want a
diet that targets your specific health problems, if you have any.

Get your vitamin levels checked because you can easily get off track with
vitamin levels when you are dieting. You must ensure that your body is
getting all the vitamins and minerals needed for good health.

Finally, have your blood pressure checked regularly, which is customary
at any doctor's visit.

With the blood panel and a blood pressure check, your doctor can tell
how you are doing. If your numbers come back and they are not within
(or moving toward) the acceptable range, that is an indicator that
something is not working.

If you know that you have been exercising faithfully, you would know that your diet is not working. Even if you are losing weight on the diet, it does not mean that your diet is addressing your health problems – and you want a diet that does.

So, if you have been on a specific diet for six months and have lost pounds and, but your glucose levels are still out of control; it is time to switch to a different diet. Even if a diet is outlined to help with a specific health issue like the **DASH Diet** that is recommended for hypertension, it may not work for everyone.

Everyone's body is different and what works for one person is not 100% guaranteed to work for another. If you started the **DASH Diet** to help with hypertension and your numbers are not dropping down into the range the doctor wants them to be, you should switch to a different diet that has proven results with high blood pressure such as **Weight Watchers.**

Weight Watchers can help lower blood pressure in some people that struggle with the problem on other diets.

Or, you may want to try a basic "close-to-nature," healthy diet with limited sodium and no alcohol like the **Flexitarian Diet**, plus adequate exercise.

Each diet is unique – just like you are. If you try one for a reasonable amount of time and do not achieve the results you want (and need), do not give up. Stop that diet and try another. With the number of healthy diets available, you are sure to find one that will work for you.

You may even want to switch up diet meal plans throughout the week! It is perfectly acceptable to try two or even more diet meal plans. Sometimes a combination diet works best. For example, you may adhere to a vegetarian diet three days a week and follow a **_Mediterranean Diet_** for the remaining four days.

To make your food preparation easier, check out my new cookbook, **_The Healthy Diet Cookbook,_** for a large collection of recipes written for seven different types of health-related diets. It can be found on Amazon.com.

Conclusion
Eat Well to Live Well

Living a healthy life is quite simple: ***Eat well to live well!***

Eating fresh, nutritious food is more important than anything else you do to ensure a healthy body and protect yourself from illness.

Listen to Your Body

Once you eliminate fast food, junk food, and processed foods from your diet and begin feeding it healthy, nutritious food every time you eat, ***your body will tell you what it needs – so, pay attention.***

Be Sure to Exercise

The body was meant to move. Continuous inactivity is dangerous. It doesn't have to be rigorous – just consistent.

Watch Your Energy Levels

Notice if there are energy lags, keep yourself hydrated, eat when you are hungry (don't eat if you are not hungry), and go to bed when you are tired (preferably near the same time every day).

Have Regular Checkups

These should be done at least once a year, possibly more if you are older or have chronic health conditions. Ask questions about your blood work and talk with your doctor about how your diet may be impacting the results.

If you are successful in implementing the steps outlined in this book at least 80% of the time, it won't be long (60 to 90 days) before you start feeling the difference that a highly-nutritious diet, regular exercise, and adequate rest can make in your life.

The Gold Standard for Healthy Eating

The experts change their minds regularly about what foods we should eat in order to stay healthy, which creates total confusion for most of us. Finally, however, there seems to be a consensus on what we should be eating to stay healthy.

It pleases me greatly that their consensus is in complete harmony with the information in this book. The following is a summary of recent findings:

YOU SHOULD EAT . . .
- Everything in moderation.
- A variety of foods that include the following:
  - Fresh fruits, but only freshly squeezed juice (never bottled or canned).
  - Lots of vegetables, which should be the largest portion on your plate.
  - Don't overlook frozen fruits and vegetables. They are flash-frozen at their peak and retain all nutrients.
  - Whole grains, beans, nuts – choose from the following: all types of nuts, dried or canned beans; plus, wheat berries, rye berries, spelt, kamut, freekah, farro, bulgur, buckwheat, oats, quinoa, barley, and brown rice.
  - Eat fish of any kind several times a week (mackerel, rainbow trout, sardines, oysters, canned tuna, and salmon are rich sources of omega-3 fatty acids).
  - Lean poultry once or twice a week.
  - Limit red meat to only a few times a month or use it in small amounts to flavor a dish of vegetables or grains.
  - Eggs in moderation.

- Milk and cheese in limited amounts - plain (unsweetened) yogurt is the best way to get dairy.
- Healthy (unsaturated) fats, in moderation, from nuts, olive oil, and other plant-based oils, avocado, and fish
- Drink lots of water and other unsweetened beverages.
- Be generous with herbs and spices to make food taste good.

YOU SHOULD NOT EAT . . .

- Sugary beverages (sodas and energy drinks)
- Trans fats
- Too much red meat, cheese, and other forms of saturated fat
- Refined carbohydrates, such as white bread, white rice, sweetened cereals, and pastries.

Know and understand your nutrients, avoid additives and added sugars, read labels, and buy foods that are in their natural, unadulterated form.

The Mediterranean way of eating has become the gold standard for healthy eating. It emphasizes plant-based foods, including everything mentioned above, plus using healthy fats such as olive oil instead of butter. With that as your guide and the information in this book, you cannot go wrong.

About the Author

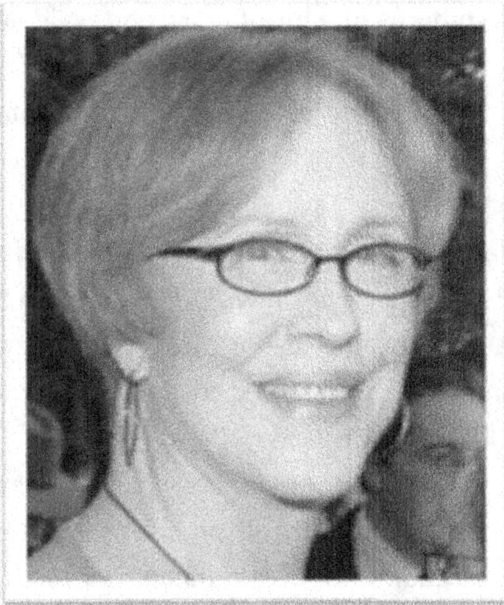

Nancy N. Wilson

All things beautiful are my passion. I enjoy anything that a masterful hand creates - writing, photography, visual arts, cooking, the human body, the human spirit, technology, our beautiful world . . . and so much more.

As a young child, I was very curious and always wanted to know why something worked and how it worked. My mother encouraged me to explore almost anything that interested me. She allowed me to take apart old clocks and radios so that I could figure out how they worked. She also gave me free rein in the kitchen to create my masterpieces of flour, sugar, spices, and anything else I could find in the cupboards.

The more I learned, the more I wanted to know, which led me quickly to the discovery of the wealth of information available in books, plus the magical journeys I could take through the power of words!

Reading became the center of my life. The town library was in the Women's Club of the little farming community that I called home. In my eyes, it was the grandest building in town - newly built, with a heavenly air-conditioner that sheltered me from the blazing heat of Arizona summers. It was my personal cocoon in which I could read the hours away.

My first adventure in writing came my senior year in high school when I decided to take a writing correspondence course, which was very forward-looking for the time. I experienced the first thrill of putting pen to paper. It was a magical new adventure! My love affair with the written word began.

Unfortunately, my affair was dealt a serious blow during my first year in college when an English professor told me that I used a lot of words but said very little. His words went to my very core and hobbled my writing confidence for several years. I continued to write, but not with the same excitement and enthusiasm that I had previously enjoyed.

It was not until many years later that everything turned around. After completing my MBA as a "mature woman" I found a position with a Leadership Development Training Company in Manhattan that required the use of three of my major passions: my insatiable curiosity of how and why things work, my love of learning through books, and my desire to write and be published.

I know, my work was not published in the traditional sense of the word, but my words were in print and people were reading them and using them to improve their professional lives. I had finally begun to realize my dream.

Now I am retired and living the dream daily. I write for many hours every day. All my work is non-fiction. Even though I love fiction, that has never been my focus and there are others who do it so much better than I. My choice has always been and will continue to be, to write about topics that interest and intrigue me and to share what I discover with my readers.

Other Books by This Author

Cookbooks

Candy Making Made Easy - Instructions and 17 Starter Recipes
Cake Making Made Easy - Instructions and 60 Cakes
Cook Ahead – Freezer to Table
The Healthy Diet Cookbook
Garden Fresh Soups and Stews
Juicing for Life – The Secret to Vibrant Health
Sweet Treats – Candy, Cookies, Cake, Ice Cream, Pudding, and Pie
Fun in the Kitchen for Tweens and Teens
Healthy Recipes for Everyone who is . . . SINGLE, ON-YOUR-OWN, and HUNGRY

Mama's Legacy Series

Seven Volumes Available

Dinner – 55 Easy Recipes (Volume I)
Breakfast and Brunch – 60 Delicious Recipes (Volume II)
Dessert – 50 Scrumptious Choices (Volume III)
Chicken – 25 Classic Dinners (Volume IV)
Mexican Favorites – 21 Traditional Recipes (Volume V)
Side Dishes – 60 Great Recipes (Volume VI)
Sauce Recipes – 50 Tasty Choices (Volume VII)

Health and Fitness

DETOX – The Master Cleanse Diet
Growing Tomatoes – Everything You Need to Know, and More
Stop Eating Yourself into an Early Grave

Business

Attitude Adjustment
Starting an Online Business
Congratulations, You Are Self-Employed

Books Written under Pseudonyms

Power Up Your Brain – Five Simple Strategies (J. J. Jackson)
Roses . . . Everything You Need to Know, and More (Susan Sumner)
Clicker Training for Dogs (Amy Ellsworth)
Making Money with Storage Unit Auctions (Bryce Cranston)

Addendum

Portion Guidelines

In order to control the amount of food you eat, you must be able to easily judge how much food is on your plate. This can be tricky because it is not easy to visualize how much equals a certain number of tablespoons, ounces, or cups. This makes serving an adequate portion challenging.

Below are some comparisons that can help you calculate healthy portions.

Basic Guidelines for Healthy Portions

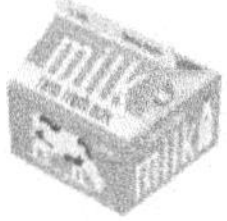

8 oz of liquid = a kid's milk carton

1 teaspoon = an average thumb from the first knuckle to the end 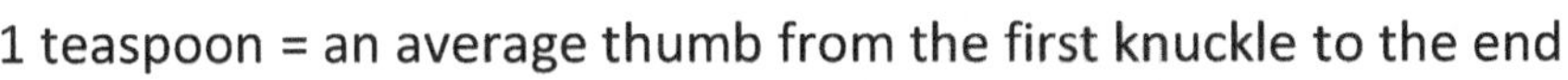

1 tablespoon = 1 poker chip 

1 oz or 2 tablespoons = 1 shot glass 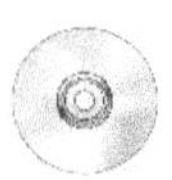

1 oz sliced deli meat = 1 CD

1½ oz of cheese = 3 gambling dice 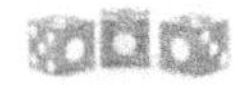

1 oz serving of meat = a matchbox 

3 oz chicken, meat, fish = a boxed deck of cards 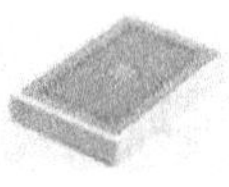

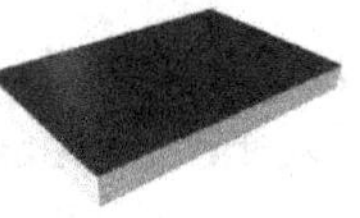

8 oz chicken meat, fish = an average paperback book

3 oz muffin or biscuit = hockey puck 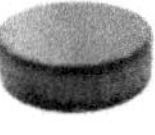

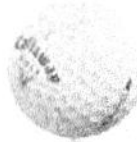

¼ cup/1oz/2 tablespoons = a golf ball

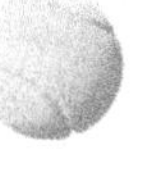

1/3 cup = a tennis ball

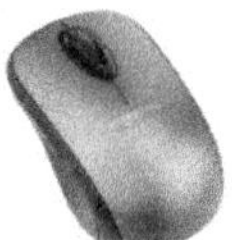

½ cup = a computer mouse

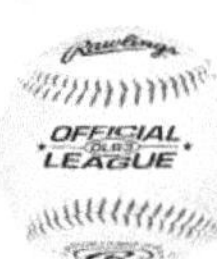

1 cup = a baseball (not softball)

Additional Examples

Meats, Fish & Nuts

3 oz lean meat of fist = deck of cards

3 oz tofu = deck of cards

2 T. peanut butter = golf ball

¼ C. pistachios = about 24 nuts

¼ C. almonds = about 23 nuts

Fruits & Vegetables

½ C. red grapes = 16

1 C. medium strawberries = 12

1 C. lettuce = baseball

1 small potato = computer mouse

1 C. baby carrots – 12

1 C. banana – 1 large

Dairy & Cheese

1 C. yogurt = baseball

½ C. ice cream = computer mouse

Breads & Grains

1 C. cereal = 1 baseball

3 C. popcorn = 3 baseballs

½ C. cooked rice = computer mouse

Fats & Oils

1 T. butter = 1 poker chip

1 T. mayo = 1 poker chip

1 C. fresh corn – 1 large ear of corn

Introspective Evaluation

The first step is to take a <u>completely honest look at yourself</u> from head to toe, inside and out – physically, mentally, and emotionally.

Answer each of the questions honestly and in as much detail, as possible.

1. How do you feel about the current state of your physical and mental health?

2. What do you really want out of life when it comes to your physical and mental health?

3. Are you content with the way you look and feel physically and mentally? ___Yes___No. Why?

4. List your daily behaviors that contribute to good health and should be continued.

5. List your daily behaviors that DO NOT contribute to good health and should be changed or eliminated completely?

6. What are three major changes you should make to be healthy and feel good . . .
    a. Physically
        1)
        2)
        3)

    b. Mentally
        1)
        2)
        3)

Where, When, and How Do You Eat?

Where do you eat on a typical day? *Do you stand, sit at a table, eat while driving or walking? Do you eat at your desk while you are working? Do you eat your meals standing up or in your car because it is faster?*

Where do you eat each of the following?
- Breakfast:
- Morning Snack:
- Lunch:
- Afternoon Snack:
- Dinner:
- Bedtime Snack:

What time of day do you eat? *Do you skip breakfast? Do you just drink coffee until noon, then eat lunch? Maybe you eat breakfast and dinner but skip lunch. Do you eat a couple of snacks in the am and pm, then have dinner? Do you have bedtime snacks?*

What time of the day do you eat each of the following:
- Breakfast:
- Morning Snack:
- Lunch:
- Afternoon Snack:
- Dinner:
- Bedtime Snack:

How do you eat? *Do you graze or feast? Do you starve and then binge? Do you enjoy food, savoring each bite, or do you eat rapidly just to get it done? Do you always eat alone, or do you eat with friends and/or family? Do you grab every available snack and gobble it down? Do you skip meals because you don't have time and then eat a candy bar in two or three bites because you are starving?*

How do you typically eat each of the following:
- Breakfast:
- Morning Snack:
- Lunch:
- Afternoon Snack:
- Dinner:
- Bedtime Snack:

What Type of Eater Are you?

Knowing the type of eater you are can be very helpful in planning your new way of eating. It will be especially useful in setting appropriate boundaries that will lead to better health. And, it may help you recognize some things you need to do to develop a healthier relationship with food. See if you can identify yourself. When it comes to types, there is always overlap, so you may see yourself in more than one.

_______***Chaotic Eater***_ – Has no routine for eating and frequently skips meals. When rushed, tend to eat on the run. They never plan-ahead, they simply grab whatever is easy and available. Have no memory of what or when they last ate.

_______***Unconscious Eater***_ – Rarely, if ever, sits down to eat. They almost always eat while doing something else - working, driving, walking, talking, reading, or watching TV. No thought is given to what they are eating – or would be hard pressed to tell you if they were hungry, or full.

_______***Emotional Eater***_ — This eater continually uses food to cope with or avoid emotions – to numb themselves from what they are feeling. They cannot stop themselves. They are aware that they eat too much, but don't think about it until after they have finished.

NOTE: If you think you may be an emotional eater, please get help. Your life could depend on it.

_______***Waste-not Eater***_ – Cannot tolerate seeing food go to waste. Always on the lookout for food deals. They always overeat when food is available in abundance such as the All-You-Can-Eat Buffet, Supersize Meal Deals, and "two-for-one" offers.

________**Do-not-offend Eater** – Cannot say no to the offer of food because it may offend or disappoint the person making the offer. They give too much power to others regarding their food choices and how much they eat rather than listening to what their bodies need.

________**Yo-Yo Eater** – This eater is always on a diet and has specific lists of "Good Food" and "Bad Food" and are always tracking what they eat or how much they eat – never listening to what their bodies are saying. They vacillate between undereating and overeating. They rarely enjoy food or the process of eating and are always worried about what they should, or should not, eat.

________**Intuitive Eater** – This type pays attention to his body and its hunger signals. They eat until they are full and don't worry about overeating. They enjoy food and trust themselves to eat well. They have no guilt about eating food they enjoy. They are conscious and mindful of the food choices, which usually are healthy choices.

The above was adapted from the book, _Intuitive Eating_.

Important Numbers

Beginning Date ______________________

Beginning Weight ______________________

Beginning BMI ______________________

Beginning Activity Level ____

Weight Goal ______________________

BMI Goal ______________________

Activity Level Goal ____

To reach your goal, it will take as long as it takes.
Patience is important.

Calorie Requirements:

Maintain Weight ______ Mild Weight Loss ______

Healthy Weight Loss ________ Extreme Weight Loss ______

Factor-in what you know about your body. According to Calculator.net, I can lose weight at 1,500/day. I know from experience that I cannot. I must eat 1,200/day to lose weight.

Weigh-ins (Quarter Check-ins are in bold):

End of Month 1 _________

End of Month 2 _________

End of Month 3 _________

Activity Level _________

End of Month 4 _________

End of Month 5 _________

End of Month 6 _________

Activity Level _________

End of Month 7 _________

End of Month 8 _________

End of Month 9 _________

Activity Level _________

End of Month 10 _________

End of Month 11 _________

End of Month 12 _________

Activity Level _________

End of Month 13 _________

End of Month 14 _________

End of Month 15 _________

Activity Level _________

End of Month 16 _________

End of Month 17 _________

End of Month 18 _________

Activity Level _________

Lessons Learned from
Tracking My Eating Habits

1. Make two lists of your food choices:

Eat in Abundance   ***Eat Occasionally***

2. How did your foods choices during the week help or hurt you?

3. What was your daily calorie intake and the average for the week?
    Was it more or less than you anticipated? How close was it to the
    calorie intake you determined should be your norm, depending
    on your goals?

4. Was there any weight variation (gain or loss)? If yes – what do you
    think contributed to the gain or loss?

5. How did you feel physically throughout the week?

6. How did you feel mentally and emotionally throughout the week?

7. How was your energy? Did it vary at all? If yes, when did it
    change?

8. Do you have any health conditions or concerns that improved or
    worsened?

Portion Control

Think for a moment about the last few meals you have eaten and answer the following questions:

What size plate do you normally use? Do you have the large dinner plates in your home that are used regularly? Or, do you have the smaller "lunch" plates?

How did you fill your plate? Was it stacked to overflowing, or was there white space showing? This is particularly a problem with the bigger plates.

Which foods took up most of the room on your plate? Meat or fatty foods like Mac & Cheese? Or, mashed potatoes smothered with butter or gravy? Were there any vegetables or whole grains? If either of those were on your plate, what was the portion size compared to the other foods?

Be honest in this evaluation. It is important to see how your typical plate looks against the health and wellness plates you plan to prepare in the future for your new way of eating.

How Often Do You Eat?

What is your preferred eating pattern?

___________ Mini-meals (Eat 5-6 times a day)

___________ Traditional three meals a day, plus snacks, when needed

___________ Do you eat breakfast ?

Why do you eat the way you do?

Do you think your current eating pattern works for you? _________ Why or why not?

Do you think it is a good choice for the future based on the healthy eating goals you now have?_________ Why or why not?

Have you considered that a different pattern may serve you better?_________ Why or why not?

Why do you eat (or not eat) breakfast?

State of Your Health

Your current state of health should be factored into your planning. The following is for informational purposes only and is not meant to be accepted as medical advice – that must come from a licensed health-care professional.

After reading through Chapter Six, answer the following questions:

1. Do you have any health issues that should be addressed in developing a healthy eating plan? If you do, what are they?

2. Are you under a doctor's care for the issues?________ What are his/her instructions regarding your diet?

3. If your goal is to lose weight, has your doctor recommended a particular diet?________ If yes, which one – and why?

4. If the answer is no, is there a diet that you would like to consider, and present to your doctor for his opinion?

5. If you have no health issues, is there a diet that you are considering for your first step – and possibly longer?

    ____

    What are the reasons you chose that plan?

How Active Are You?

Now that you have studied the different levels of activity in Chapter Eight, answer the following questions:

1. Which level describes your physical activity the best? ________________

2. How much and what type of activity to you get on a weekly basis?

3. Which level is your goal? ________________________________

4. How are you going to work up to that level?

5. How many hours a day do you spend sitting? ______________ Do you take regular stand-up or walking breaks? __________ How many per day ____________? How long is each break?__________.

6. Create a plan for how you are going to improve your daily activity.